DIABETIC
COOKING

Publications International, Ltd.

Favorite Brand Name Recipes at www.fbnr.com

Pictured on the front cover *(clockwise from top left):* Thai-Style Pork Kabobs *(page 32),* Apricot Biscotti *(page 88),* Mixed Berry Cheesecake *(page 90),* Ravioli with Tomato Pesto *(page 22),* Cream Cheese Brownie Royale *(page 80),* Italian Crouton Salad *(page 34)* and Apple-Cranberry Crescent Cookies *(page 91).*

Pictured on the back cover *(clockwise from top left):* Scrambled Egg Burrito *(page 16),* Silly Spaghetti Casserole *(page 52),* Blackberry Sorbet *(page 86)* and Chili Beef & Red Pepper Fajita with Chipotle Salsa *(page 40).*

ISBN: 1-4127-2029-X

Manufactured in China.

8 7 6 5 4 3 2 1

Nutritional Analysis: The nutritional information that appears with each recipe was submitted in part by the participating companies and associations. Every effort has been made to check the accuracy of these numbers. However, because numerous variables account for a wide range of values for certain foods, nutritive analyses in this book should be considered approximate.

Microwave Cooking: Microwave ovens vary in wattage. Use the cooking times as guidelines and check for doneness before adding more time.

Preparation/Cooking Times: Preparation times are based on the approximate amount of time required to assemble the recipe before cooking, baking, chilling or serving. These times include preparation steps such as measuring, chopping and mixing. The fact that some preparations and cooking can be done simultaneously is taken into account. Preparation of optional ingredients and serving suggestions is not included.

table of
contents

introduction

Whether you or someone close to you has recently been diagnosed with diabetes or has been living with it for years, don't be discouraged. We now know more about diabetes than ever before, and research is constantly providing us with information on new and better ways of managing it. Today people with diabetes are living long, happy and healthy lives.

No Foods Are Forbidden

In the past, people with diabetes were told to monitor the amount of sugar in every food they ate. While it used to be thought that simple sugar, such as the type in cake and cookies, caused a larger rise in blood glucose than other types of carbohydrates, research has proven otherwise. Today the focus has shifted away from sugar to focus on the total amount of carbohydrates consumed throughout the day. Better known as "Carbohydrate Counting," this system is much more flexible than the older, more rigid Exchange System.

Instead of telling patients what foods to avoid, health professionals are now instructing them on healthy eating and foods to choose. Registered dietitians and certified diabetes educators everywhere are working with patients, instructing them on ways to include a wide variety of foods—even sugary ones in moderation—in their meal plans. Because this system, "Carbohydrate Counting," is the one being taught by so many professionals today, the amount of sugar is not included with the nutritional analyses for the recipes in this book. You will, however, find the total amount of carbohydrates and the exchange information given for each recipe.

If you haven't already, ask your medical doctor or endocrinologist to refer you to a registered dietitian or a certified diabetes educator. Either of these professionals will talk with you and help you better understand your diabetes and instruct you on ways to control it. They will be able to calculate the number of servings of carbohydrates you need each day and can work with you to devise a meal plan that best fits your lifestyle.

It's All About Balance

Goals for healthful eating are based on total foods consumed throughout the day or over a period of time, instead of only on individual foods. A food might be high in carbohydrates, but if other foods eaten throughout the day are adjusted to meet a person's total suggested carbohydrate intake, the single high-carbohydrate food will not likely pose a problem. Because of this, a range of healthful recipes are included within this book. Some of the recipes are higher in sodium; some are higher in fat; and some are higher in carbohydrates or cholesterol. Moderation, portion sizes and planning are keys to success with any healthful eating plan.

A diagnosis of diabetes brings about a whole new way living. The satisfying recipes in this book are intended to help make this transition as smooth as possible. Let them be your guide to providing delicious and nutritious meals!

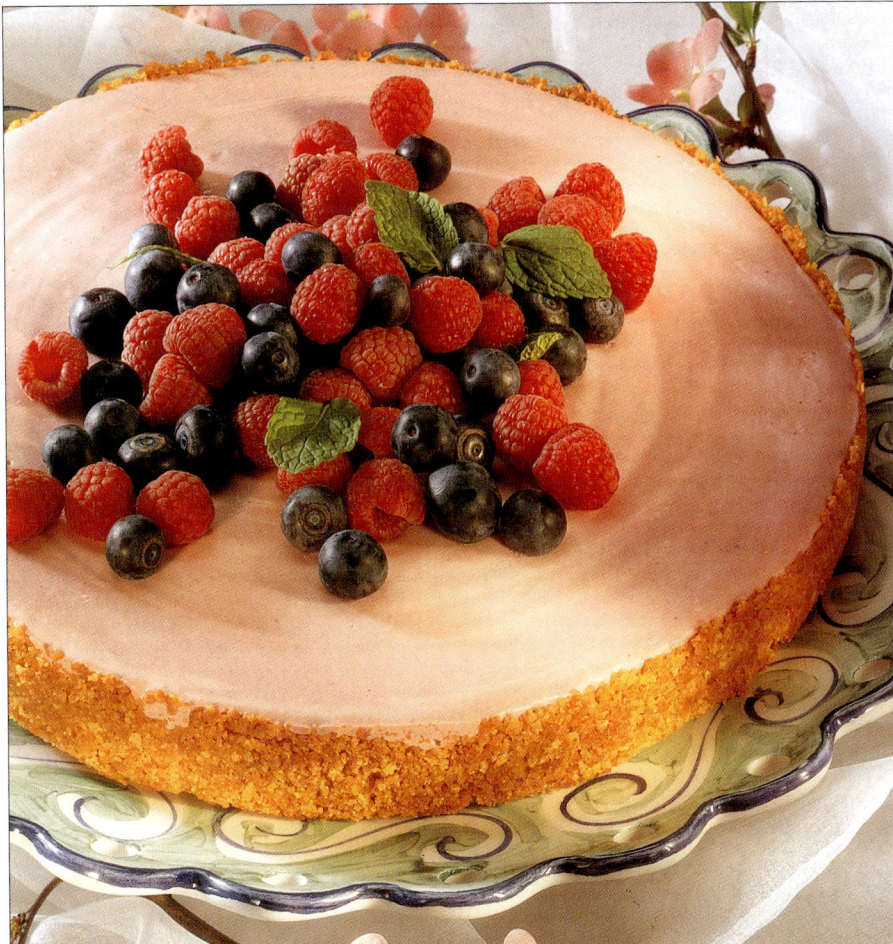

Mixed Berry Cheesecake *(recipe on page 90)*

breakfast delights

Farmstand Frittata

Makes 4 servings

Nonstick cooking spray
½ cup chopped onion
1 medium red bell pepper, seeded and cut into thin strips
1 cup broccoli florets, blanched and drained
1 cup cooked, quartered unpeeled red potatoes
1 cup cholesterol-free egg substitute
6 egg whites
1 tablespoon chopped fresh parsley
½ teaspoon salt
¼ teaspoon black pepper
½ cup (2 ounces) shredded reduced-fat Cheddar cheese

1. Spray large nonstick ovenproof skillet with cooking spray; heat over medium heat until hot. Add onion and bell pepper; cook and stir 3 minutes or until crisp-tender. Add broccoli and potatoes; cook and stir 1 to 2 minutes or until hot.

2. Whisk together egg substitute, egg whites, parsley, salt and black pepper in medium bowl. Pour over vegetables. Cover; cook 10 to 12 minutes or until egg mixture is set.

3. Meanwhile, preheat broiler. Top frittata with cheese. Broil 4 inches from heat 1 minute or until cheese is melted. Cut into four wedges.

Nutrients per serving: 1 Frittata wedge (¼ of total recipe)
Calories: 163, **Calories from Fat:** 12%, **Total Fat:** 2g,
Saturated Fat: 1g, **Cholesterol:** 8mg, **Sodium:** 686mg,
Carbohydrate: 19g, **Fiber:** 2g, **Protein:** 17g

Dietary Exchange: 1 Starch, 2 Meat

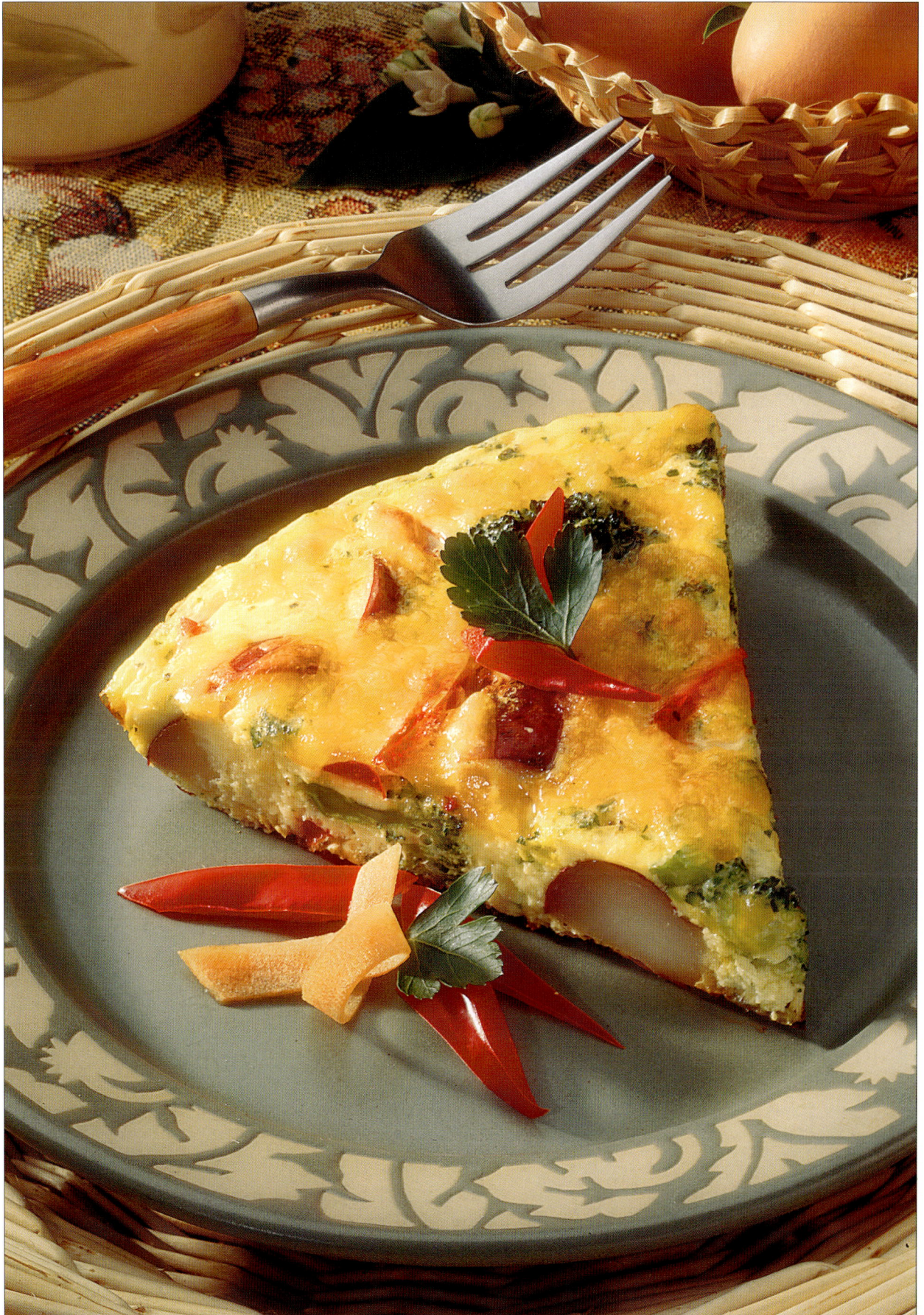

Farmstand Frittata

English Muffin Breakfast Sandwiches

Makes 4 servings (1 muffin half each)

- 2 English muffins, split into halves and toasted
- 2 tablespoons plain nonfat yogurt
- 1 tablespoon spicy brown or Dijon mustard
- ½ teaspoon dried tarragon or basil leaves
- 4 slices Canadian bacon
- 4 large tomato slices (about ¼-inch thick)
- 2 slices (1 ounce each) reduced-fat Swiss cheese, cut crosswise into halves *or* 1 cup (4 ounces) shredded part-skim mozzarella cheese
- 4 poached eggs, kept warm
- Paprika (optional)

1. Preheat broiler.

2. Place muffin halves on baking sheet or broiler pan.

3. Combine yogurt, mustard and tarragon in small bowl; stir until well blended. Spread ¼ of yogurt mixture evenly over each muffin half. Top each muffin half with Canadian bacon and tomato slice.

4. Top each tomato slice with cheese slice half. Place under broiler about 4 inches from heat source; broil 1 minute or until cheese begins to brown slightly. Top with poached eggs. Sprinkle with paprika, if desired.

Nutrients per serving:
Calories: 233, Calories from Fat: 35%, Total Fat: 9g, Saturated Fat: 3g, Cholesterol: 233mg, Sodium: 836mg, Carbohydrate: 17g, Fiber: 1g, Protein: 18g

Dietary Exchange: 1 Starch, 2½ Meat, ½ Fat

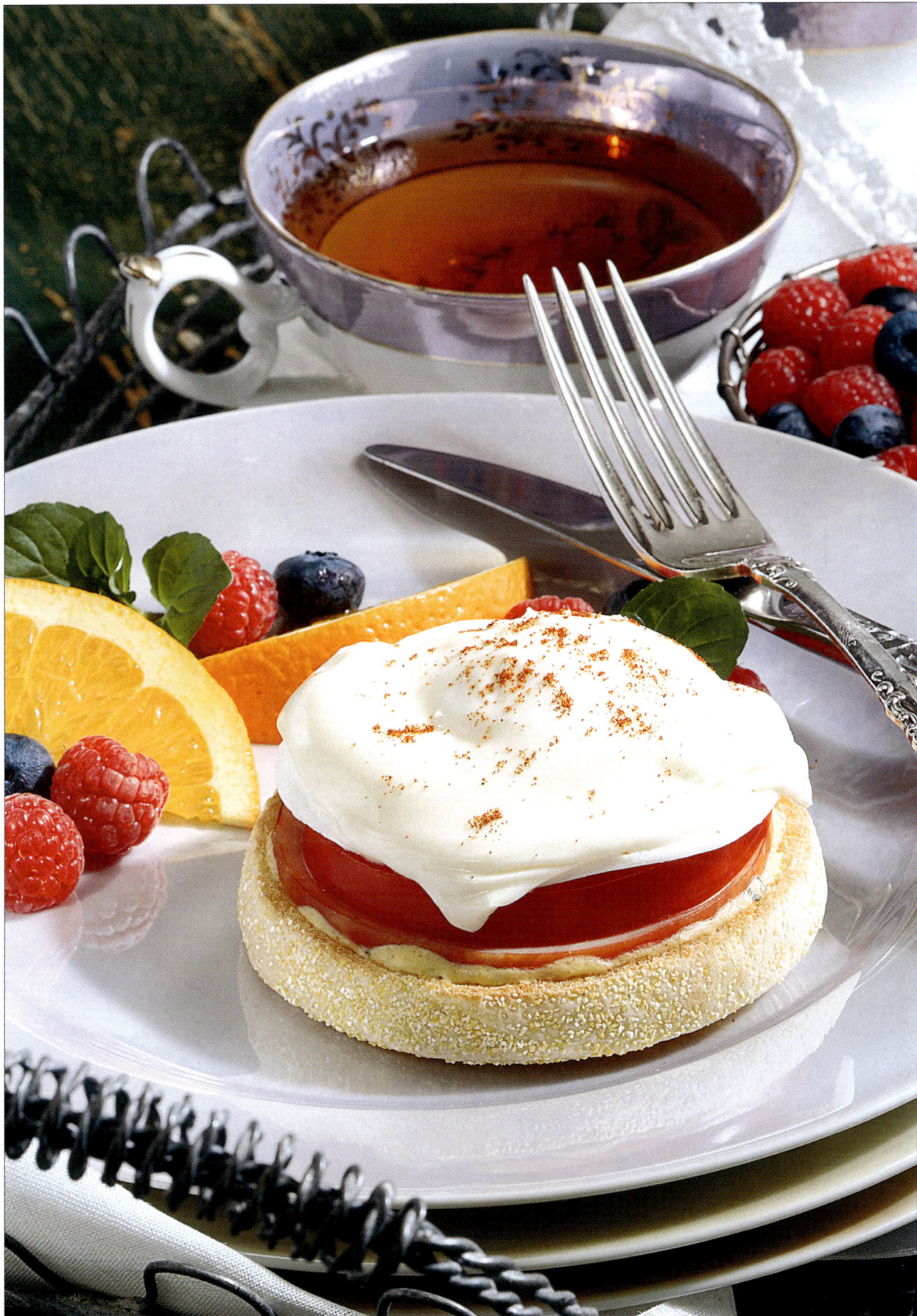

English Muffin Breakfast Sandwich

Cornmeal Scones

Makes 16 servings

½ **cup dried currants**
1 **cup warm water**
1⅓ **cups all-purpose flour**
⅔ **cup cornmeal**
½ **cup plus 1 teaspoon sugar, divided**
1½ **teaspoons baking powder**
½ **teaspoon baking soda**
¼ **teaspoon salt**
¼ **cup (½ stick) cold margarine, cut into 4 pieces**
¼ **cup plain nonfat yogurt**
3 **tablespoons fat-free (skim) milk**
1 **egg, lightly beaten**
1 **egg white, lightly beaten**

1. Preheat oven to 375°F. Lightly spray baking sheet with nonstick cooking spray; set aside. Place currants in small mixing bowl. Add water; let stand 10 minutes. Drain and discard water.

2. Combine flour, cornmeal, ½ cup sugar, baking powder, baking soda and salt in large mixing bowl. Cut margarine into flour mixture with pastry blender or 2 knives until mixture resembles coarse crumbs. Stir in currants.

3. Combine yogurt, milk and whole egg in small bowl. Add to flour mixture, stirring just until dry ingredients are moistened. Turn out dough onto lightly floured surface; knead 5 or 6 times. Shape dough into 8-inch round. Place on baking sheet. Brush with egg white; sprinkle with remaining 1 teaspoon sugar. Cut into 8 wedges. Bake 20 minutes or until lightly browned. Cool on wire rack. Cut each wedge in half.

Nutrients per serving: 1 Scone (1⁄16 of total recipe)
Calories: 132, **Calories from Fat:** 23%, **Total Fat:** 3g,
Saturated Fat: 1g, **Cholesterol:** 13mg, **Sodium:** 170mg,
Carbohydrate: 22g, **Fiber:** 1g, **Protein:** 3g

Dietary Exchange: 1½ Starch, ½ Fat

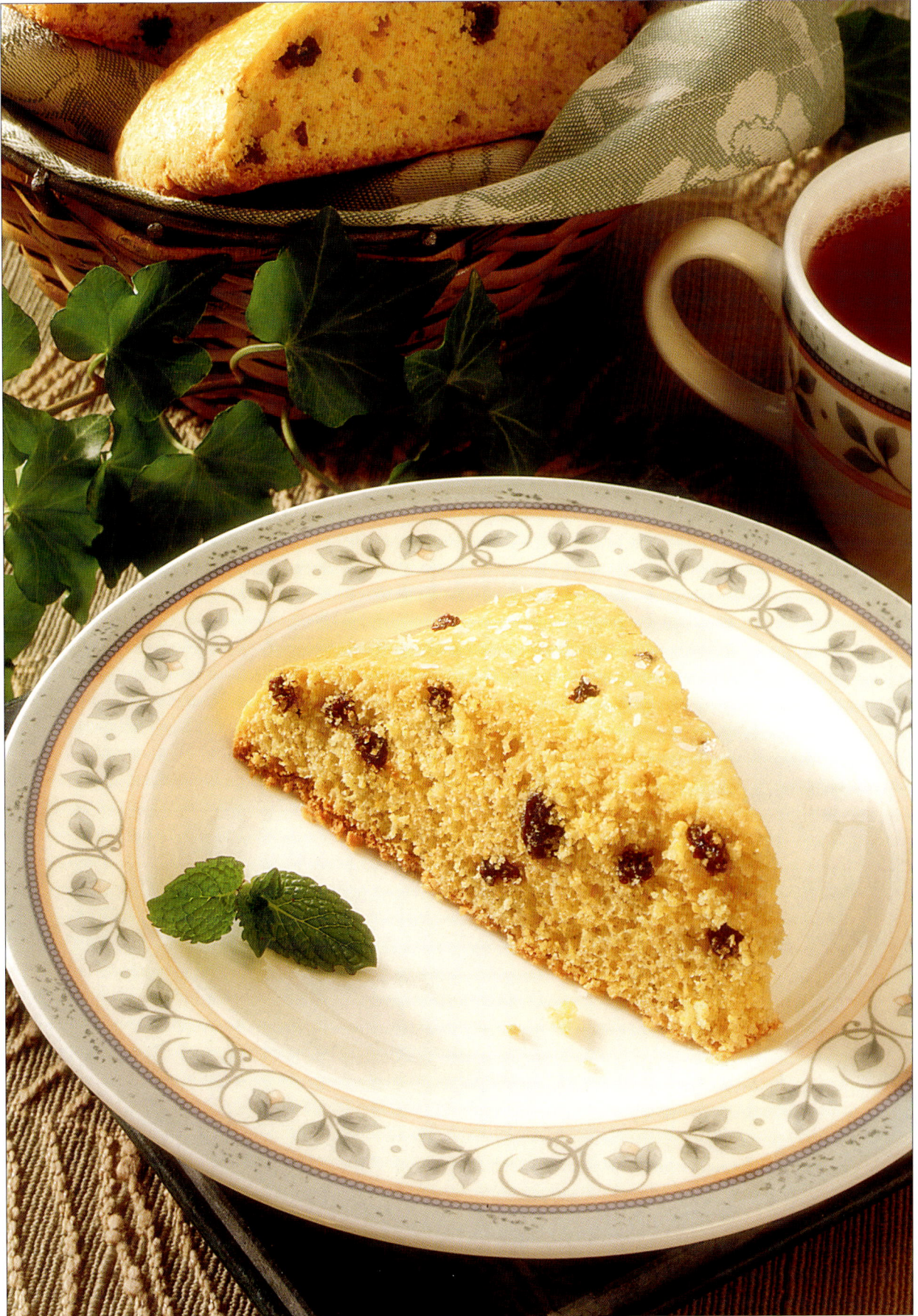

Cornmeal Scones

breakfastdelights

Mini Vegetable Quiches

Makes 8 servings

- 2 **cups cut-up vegetables (bell peppers, broccoli, zucchini and/or carrots)**
- 2 **tablespoons chopped green onions**
- 2 **tablespoons FLEISCHMANN'S® Original Margarine**
- 4 **(8-inch) flour tortillas, each cut into 8 triangles**
- 1 **cup EGG BEATERS® Healthy Real Egg Product**
- 1 **cup fat-free (skim) milk**
- ½ **teaspoon dried basil leaves**

In medium nonstick skillet, over medium-high heat, sauté vegetables and green onions in margarine until tender.

Arrange 4 tortilla pieces in each of 8 (6-ounce) greased custard cups or ramekins, placing points of tortilla pieces at center of bottom of each cup and pressing lightly to form shape of cup. Divide vegetable mixture evenly among cups. In small bowl, combine Egg Beaters®, milk and basil. Pour evenly over vegetable mixture. Place cups on baking sheet. Bake at 375°F for 20 to 25 minutes or until puffed and knife inserted into centers comes out clean. Let stand 5 minutes before serving.

Nutrients per serving: 1 Quiche
Calories: 115, **Calories from Fat:** 30%, **Total Fat:** 4g,
Saturated Fat: 1g, **Cholesterol:** 1mg, **Sodium:** 184mg,
Carbohydrate: 14g, **Fiber:** 1g, **Protein:** 6g

Dietary Exchange: ½ Starch, 2 Vegetable, ½ Fat

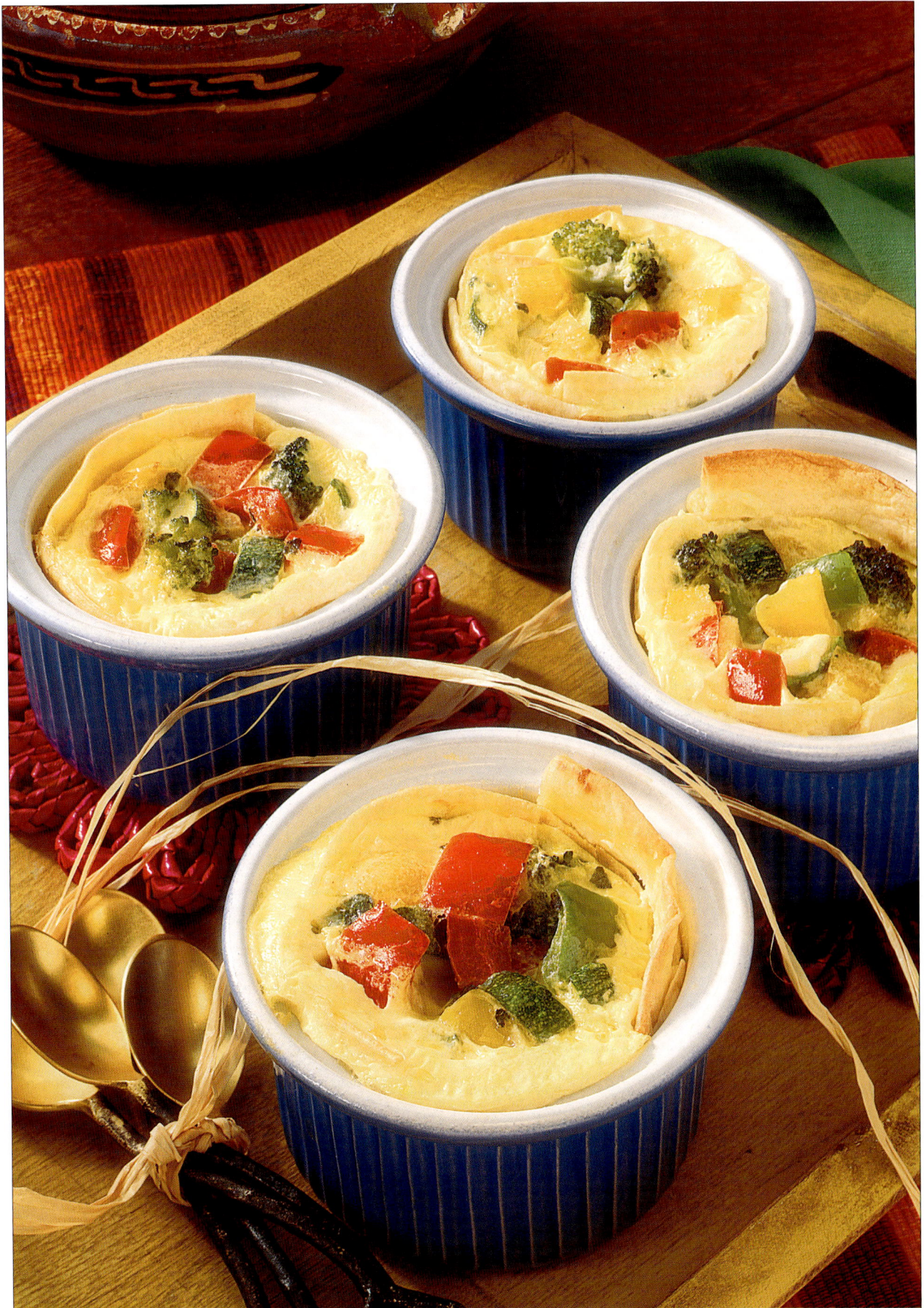

Mini Vegetable Quiches

Scrambled Egg Burritos

Makes 4 servings

    Nonstick cooking spray
1 **red bell pepper, chopped**
5 **green onions, sliced**
½ **teaspoon red pepper flakes**
1 **cup cholesterol-free egg substitute *or* 8 egg whites**
1 **tablespoon chopped fresh cilantro or parsley**
4 **(8-inch) flour tortillas**
½ **cup (2 ounces) shredded low-sodium reduced-fat Monterey Jack cheese**
⅓ **cup salsa**

1. Spray medium nonstick skillet with cooking spray. Heat over medium heat until hot. Add bell pepper, green onions and red pepper flakes. Cook and stir 3 minutes or until vegetables are crisp-tender.

2. Add egg substitute to vegetables. Reduce heat to low. Cook and stir 3 minutes or until set. Sprinkle with cilantro.

3. Stack tortillas and wrap in paper towels. Microwave at HIGH 1 minute or until tortillas are hot.

4. Place ¼ egg mixture on each tortilla. Sprinkle with 2 tablespoons cheese. Fold sides over to enclose filling. Serve with salsa.

Prep and Cook Time: 18 minutes

Nutrients per serving: 1 Burrito with 1 tablespoon plus 1 teaspoon salsa
Calories: 186, **Calories from Fat:** 20%, **Total Fat:** 4g,
Saturated Fat: 1g, **Cholesterol:** 6mg, **Sodium:** 423mg,
Carbohydrate: 23g, **Fiber:** 1g, **Protein:** 14g

Dietary Exchange: 1 Starch, 1 Vegetable, 1½ Meat

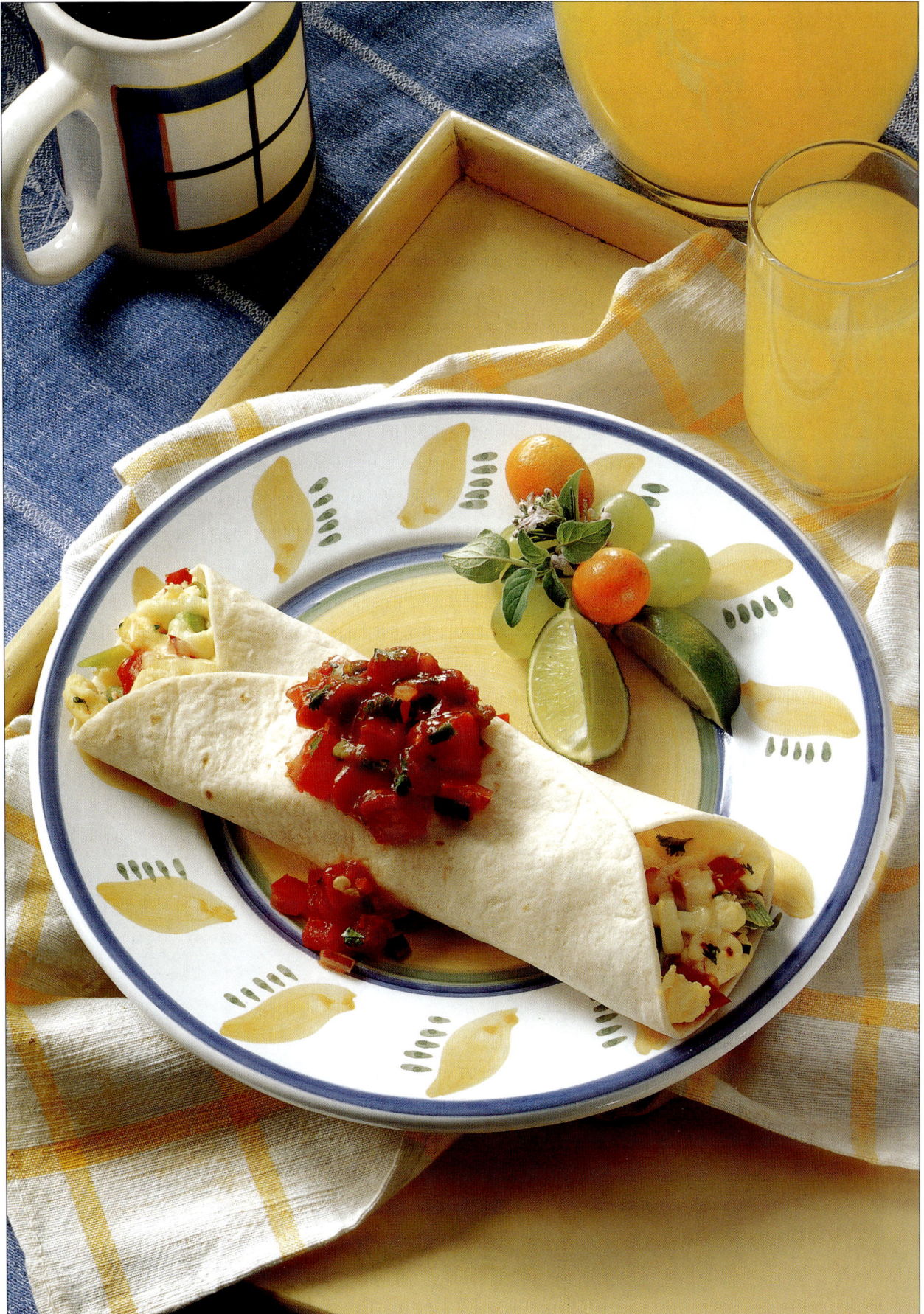

Scrambled Egg Burrito

breakfastdelights

Sausage and Red Pepper Strata

Makes 4 servings

Nonstick cooking spray
6 ounces reduced-fat breakfast bulk pork sausage
½ teaspoon dried oregano leaves
¼ teaspoon red pepper flakes (optional)
4 slices day-old French bread, cut into ½-inch pieces
½ medium red bell pepper, finely chopped
¼ cup chopped parsley
1 cup cholesterol-free egg substitute
1 cup evaporated skimmed milk
1 teaspoon Dijon mustard
¼ teaspoon black pepper
½ cup (2 ounces) shredded reduced-fat sharp Cheddar cheese

1. Spray medium nonstick skillet with cooking spray; heat over medium-high heat. Add sausage, oregano and red pepper flakes, if desired. Cook until browned. Drain on paper towels.

2. Spray 8-inch square baking dish with cooking spray. Line bottom of pan with bread. Sprinkle sausage evenly over bread; top with bell pepper and parsley.

3. Combine egg substitute, milk, mustard and black pepper in medium bowl; whisk until well blended. Pour egg mixture evenly over sausage. Cover tightly with foil and refrigerate overnight.

4. Preheat oven to 350°F. Bake, covered tightly, 55 minutes. Remove foil. Sprinkle with cheese and bake 5 minutes or until cheese is melted.

Nutrients per serving:
Calories: 298, **Calories from Fat:** 36%, **Total Fat:** 12g, **Saturated Fat:** 2g, **Cholesterol:** 43mg, **Sodium:** 719mg, **Carbohydrate:** 23g, **Fiber:** 1g, **Protein:** 25g

Dietary Exchange: 1 Starch, ½ Milk, 2 Meat, ½ Fat

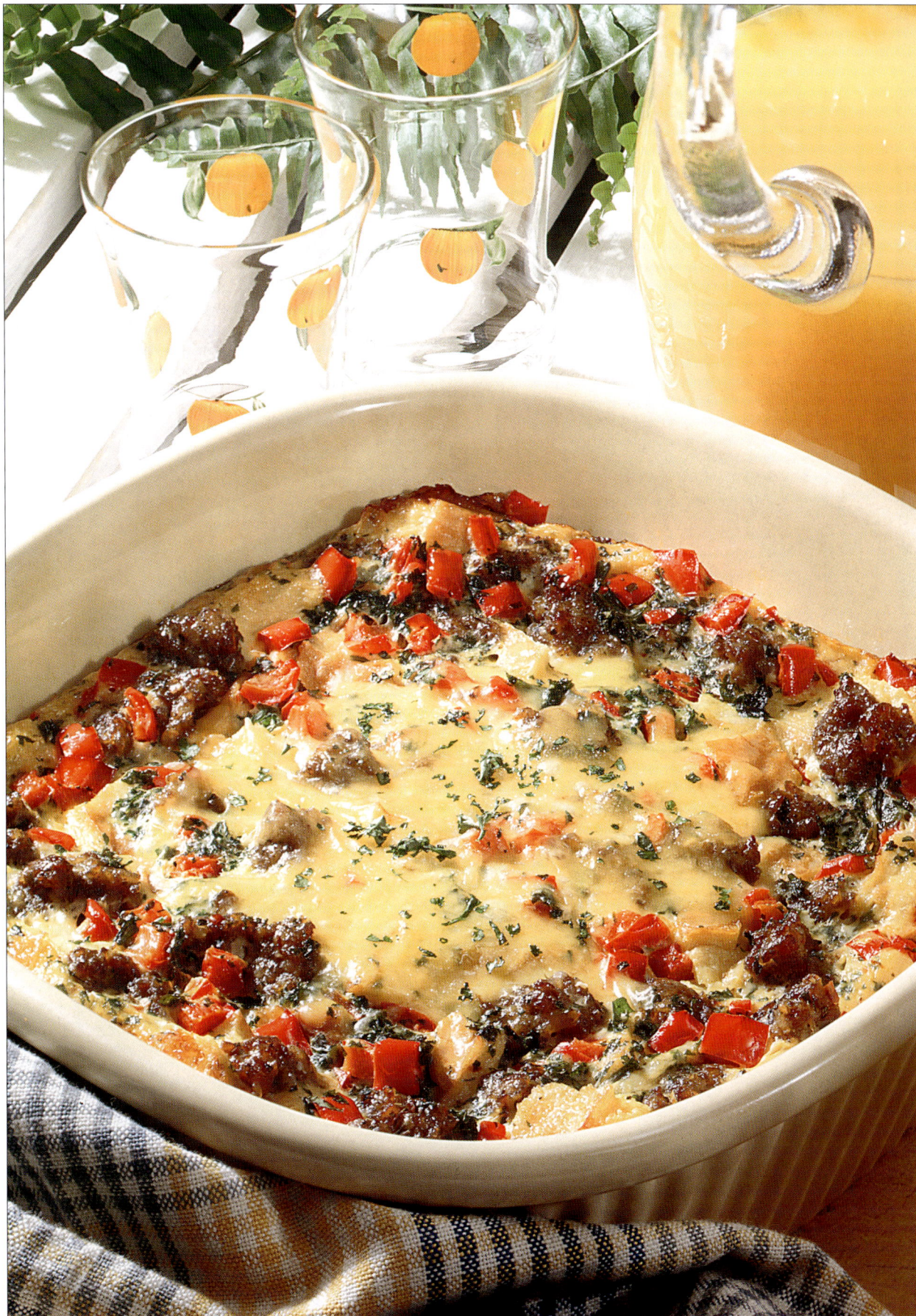

Sausage and Red Pepper Strata

breakfastdelights

Potato & Onion Frittata

Makes 2 servings

- 1 **small baking potato, peeled, halved and sliced ⅛ inch thick (about ½ cup)**
- ¼ **cup chopped onion**
- 1 **clove garlic, minced**
  Dash ground black pepper
- 1 **tablespoon FLEISCHMANN'S® Original Margarine**
- 1 **cup EGG BEATERS® Healthy Real Egg Product**

In 8-inch nonstick skillet, over medium-high heat, sauté potato, onion, garlic and pepper in margarine until tender. Pour Egg Beaters® evenly into skillet over potato mixture. Cook, without stirring, for 5 to 6 minutes or until cooked on bottom and almost set on top. Carefully turn frittata; cook for 1 to 2 minutes more or until done. Slide onto serving platter; cut into wedges to serve.

Prep Time: 5 minutes
Cook Time: 15 minutes

Nutrients per serving: 1 Frittata wedge (½ of total recipe)
Calories: 179, **Calories from Fat:** 25%, **Total Fat:** 5g, **Saturated Fat:** 1g, **Cholesterol:** 0mg, **Sodium:** 276mg, **Carbohydrate:** 19g, **Fiber:** 2g, **Protein:** 14g

Dietary Exchange: 1 Starch, 1 Meat, 1 Fat

Brunch Strata

Makes 6 servings

  1 can (10¾ ounces) reduced-fat condensed cream of celery soup, undiluted
  2 cups cholesterol-free egg substitute *or* 8 eggs
  1 cup fat-free (skim) milk
  1 can (4 ounces) sliced mushrooms (optional)
  ¼ cup sliced green onions
  1 teaspoon dry mustard
  ½ teaspoon salt (optional)
  ¼ teaspoon black pepper
  6 slices reduced-fat white bread, cut into 1-inch cubes
  4 links reduced-fat precooked breakfast sausage, thinly sliced

1. Preheat oven to 350°F. Spray 2-quart baking dish with nonstick cooking spray; set aside.

2. Combine soup, egg substitute, milk, mushrooms, if desired, green onions, mustard, salt, if desired, and pepper in medium bowl; mix well.

3. Combine bread cubes, sausage and soup mixture in prepared baking dish; toss to coat. Bake 35 to 40 minutes or until set. Garnish as desired.

Nutrients per serving: 1 cup
Calories: 155, **Calories from Fat:** 12%, **Total Fat:** 2g,
Saturated Fat: 1g, **Cholesterol:** 8mg, **Sodium:** 642mg,
Carbohydrate: 20g, **Fiber:** 3g, **Protein:** 15g

Dietary Exchange: 1 Starch, 2 Meat

main dish mania

Ravioli with Tomato Pesto

Makes 2 servings

- 4 ounces frozen cheese ravioli
- 1¼ cups coarsely chopped plum tomatoes
- ¼ cup fresh basil leaves
- 2 teaspoons pine nuts
- 2 teaspoons olive oil
- ¼ teaspoon salt
- ⅛ teaspoon black pepper
- 1 tablespoon grated Parmesan cheese

1. Cook ravioli according to package directions; drain.

2. Meanwhile, combine tomatoes, basil, pine nuts, oil, salt and pepper in food processor. Process using on/off pulsing action just until ingredients are chopped. Serve over ravioli. Top with cheese.

Nutrients per serving:
Calories: 175, **Calories from Fat:** 34%, **Total Fat:** 10g,
Saturated Fat: 2g, **Cholesterol:** 59mg, **Sodium:** 459mg,
Carbohydrate: 20g, **Fiber:** 3g, **Protein:** 10g

Dietary Exchange: 1 Starch, 1 Vegetable, 1 Meat, ½ Fat

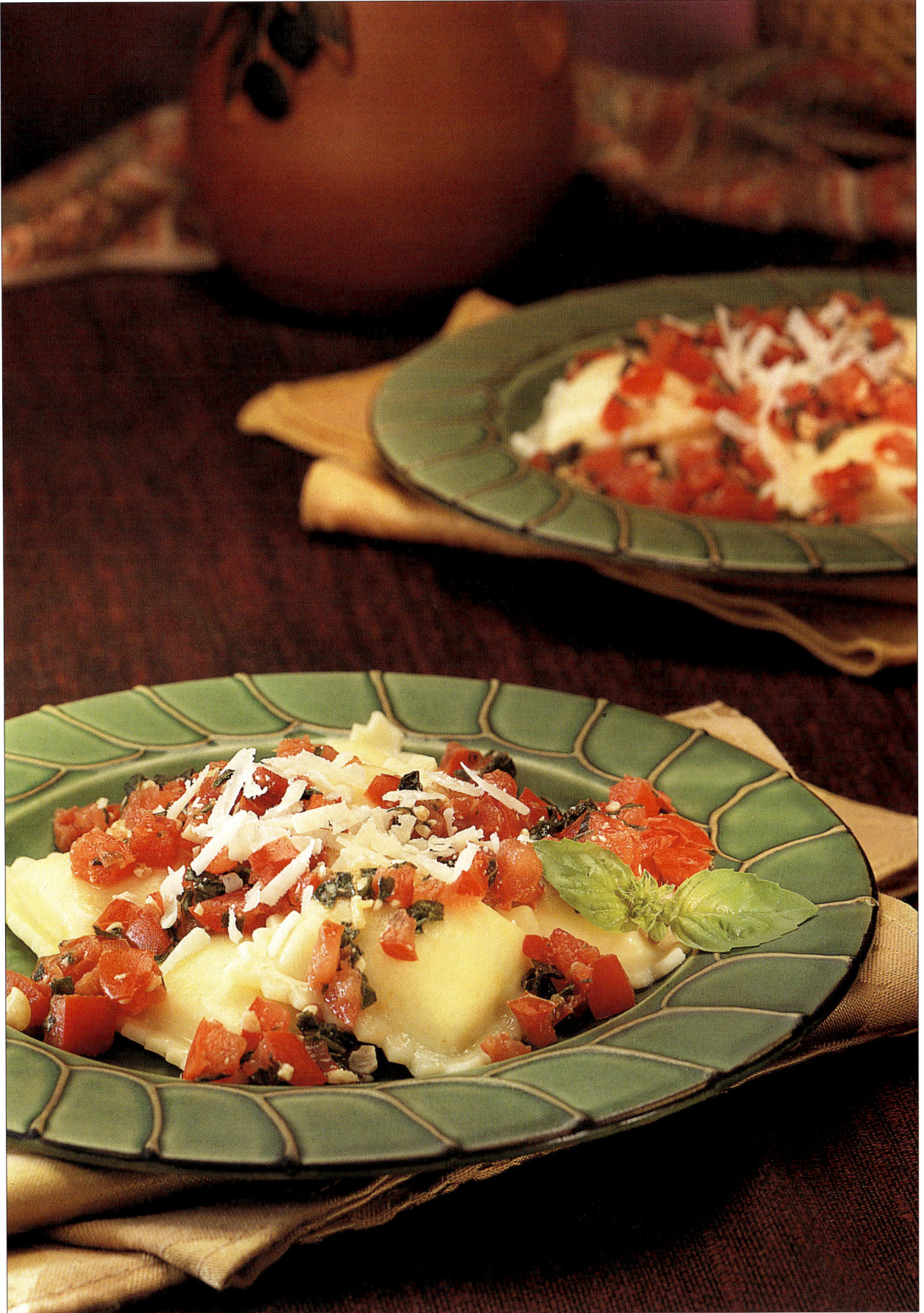
Ravioli with Tomato Pesto

Gingered Chicken with Vegetables

Makes 4 servings

- 2 **tablespoons vegetable oil, divided**
- 1 **pound boneless skinless chicken breasts, cut into thin strips**
- 1 **cup red pepper strips**
- 1 **cup sliced fresh mushrooms**
- 16 **fresh pea pods, cut in half crosswise**
- ½ **cup sliced water chestnuts**
- ¼ **cup sliced green onions**
- 1 **tablespoon grated fresh gingerroot**
- 1 **large clove garlic, crushed**
- ⅔ **cup reduced-fat, reduced-sodium chicken broth**
- 2 **tablespoons EQUAL® SPOONFUL***
- 2 **tablespoons light soy sauce**
- 4 **teaspoons cornstarch**
- 2 **teaspoons dark sesame oil**
- **Salt and pepper to taste**

*May substitute 3 packets Equal® sweetener.

• Heat 1 tablespoon vegetable oil in large skillet over medium-high heat. Stir-fry chicken until no longer pink; remove chicken from skillet. Heat remaining 1 tablespoon vegetable oil in skillet. Add bell peppers, mushrooms, pea pods, water chestnuts, green onions, ginger and garlic to skillet. Stir-fry mixture 3 to 4 minutes until vegetables are crisp-tender.

• Meanwhile, combine chicken broth, Equal®, soy sauce, cornstarch and sesame oil until smooth. Stir into skillet mixture. Cook over medium heat until thick and clear. Stir in chicken; heat through. Season with salt and pepper to taste.

• Serve over hot cooked rice, if desired.

Nutrients per serving:
Calories: 263, **Calories from Fat:** 38%, **Total Fat:** 11g,
Saturated Fat: 1g, **Cholesterol:** 66mg, **Sodium:** 411mg,
Carbohydrate: 11g, **Fiber:** 2g, **Protein:** 29g

Dietary Exchange: 2 Vegetable, 4 Meat

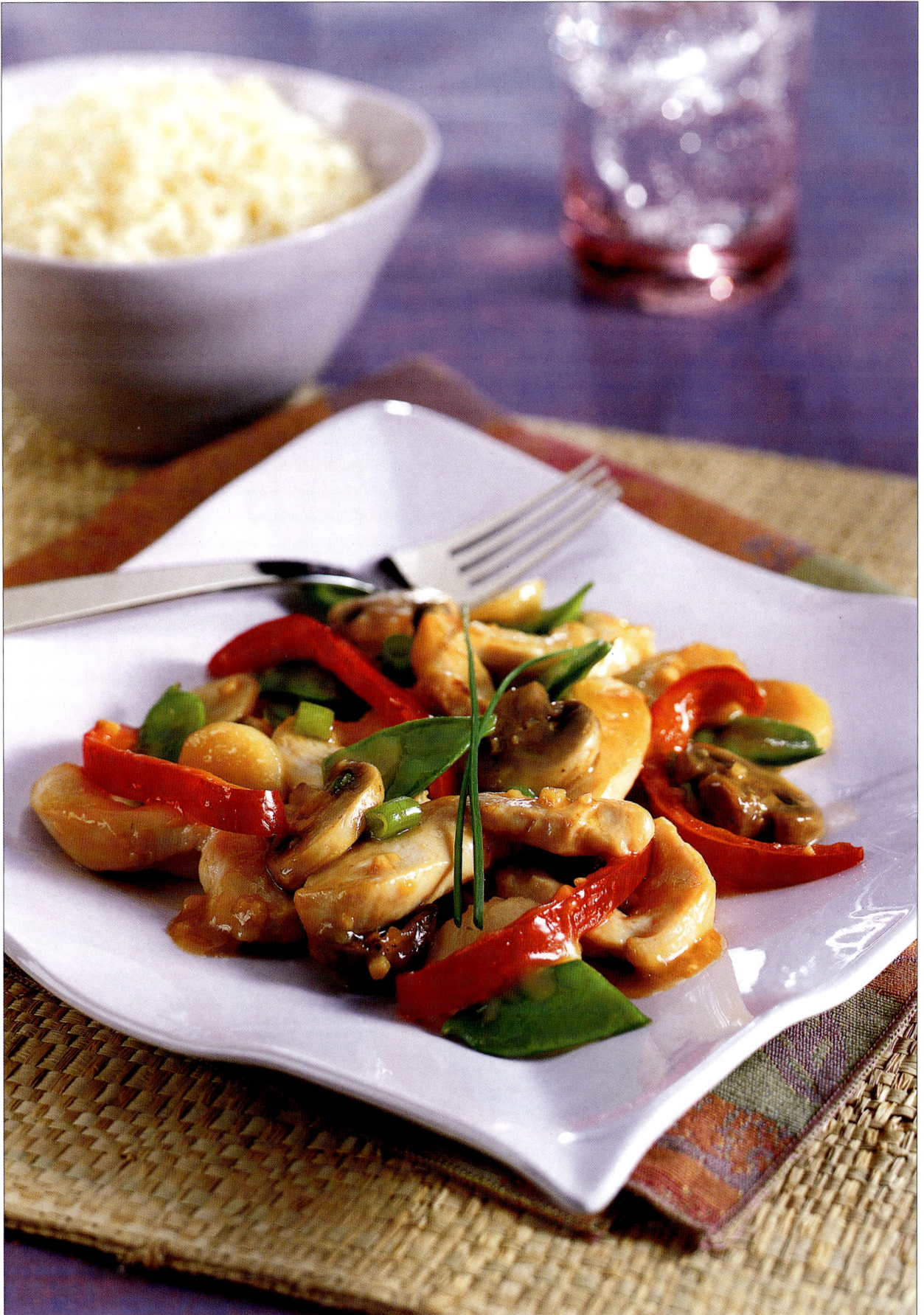

Gingered Chicken with Vegetables

Sirloin with Sweet Caramelized Onions

Makes 4 servings

    Nonstick cooking spray
1 medium onion, very thinly sliced
1 boneless beef top sirloin steak (about 1 pound)
¼ cup water
2 tablespoons Worcestershire sauce
1 tablespoon sugar

1. Lightly coat 12-inch skillet with cooking spray; heat over high heat until hot. Add onion; cook and stir 4 minutes or until browned. Remove from skillet and set aside. Wipe out skillet with paper towel.

2. Coat same skillet with cooking spray; heat until hot. Add beef; cook 10 to 13 minutes for medium-rare to medium, turning once. Remove from heat and transfer to cutting board; let stand 3 minutes before slicing.

3. Meanwhile, return skillet to high heat until hot; add onion, water, Worcestershire sauce and sugar. Cook 30 to 45 seconds or until most liquid has evaporated.

4. Thinly slice beef on the diagonal and serve with onions.

Nutrients per serving:
Calories: 159, **Calories from Fat:** 28%, **Total Fat:** 5g,
Saturated Fat: 2g, **Cholesterol:** 60mg, **Sodium:** 118mg,
Carbohydrate: 7g, **Fiber:** 1g, **Protein:** 21g

Dietary Exchange: 3 Meat

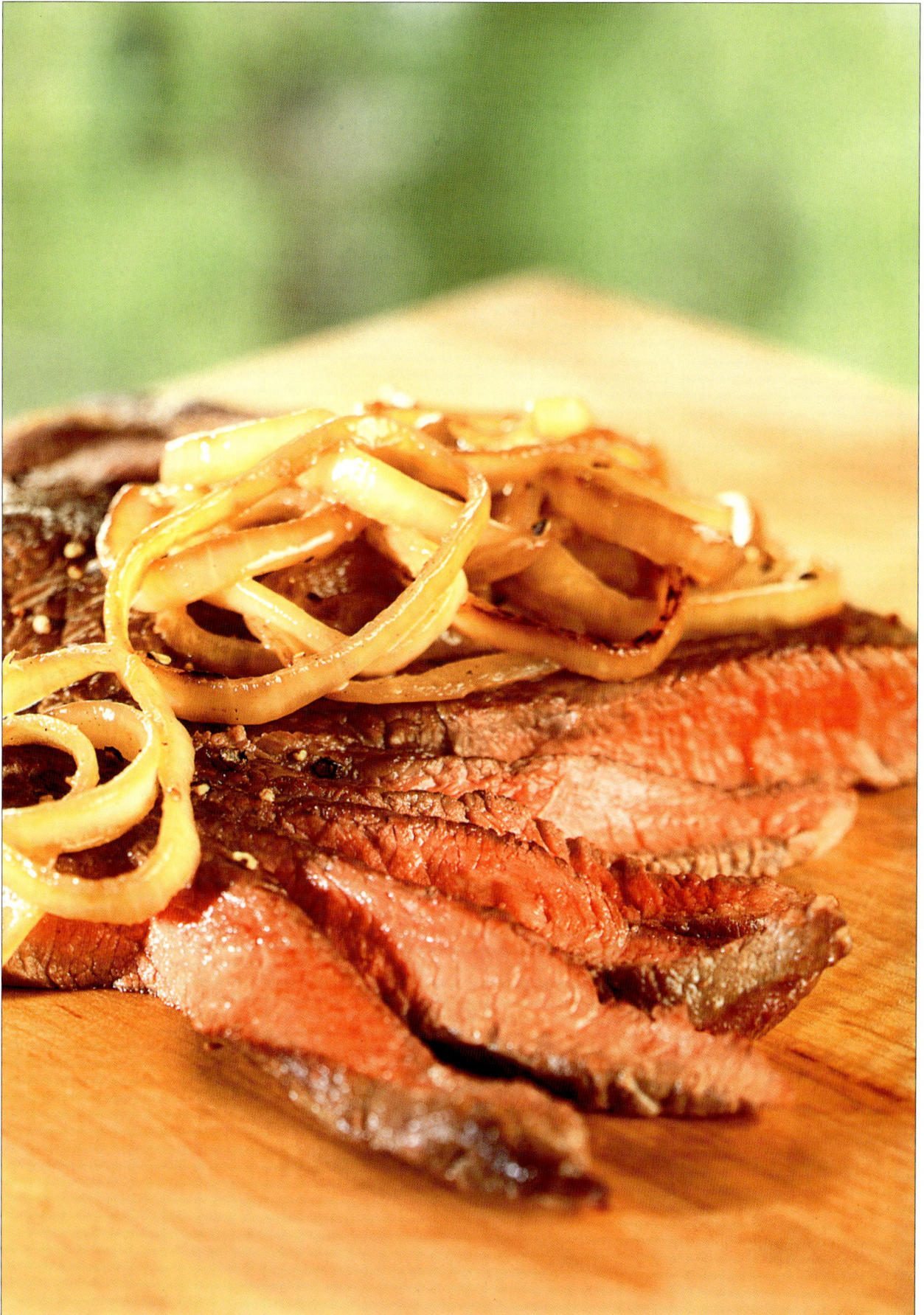

Sirloin with Sweet Caramelized Onions

Chicken with Spinach and Celery-Potato Hash

Makes 4 servings

- 1 package (16-ounces) refrigerated precooked fat-free hash browns
- 1 package (8 ounces) ready-to-use celery sticks *or* 3 ribs celery, thinly sliced
- 3 teaspoons olive oil, divided
- 12 chicken tenders (about 1 pound)
- ½ teaspoon dried thyme leaves
- ¼ teaspoon white pepper
- ¼ cup water
- 2 packages (5 ounces each) ready-to-use baby spinach

1. Mix hash browns and celery together in large bowl.

2. Heat half the oil in large nonstick skillet over medium-high heat. Add hash brown mixture; cook about 10 minutes, stirring occasionally, until mixture begins to brown. Reduce heat and continue cooking about 10 more minutes until hash is browned but not burned.

3. Heat remaining oil in 12-inch nonstick skillet over medium-high heat. Add chicken tenders. Sprinkle with thyme and white pepper. Cook about 2 to 3 minutes on each side or until chicken is no longer pink. Remove and keep warm.

4. To same skillet, add water and spinach. Cover; steam about 3 minutes, stirring once.

5. To serve, divide spinach, hash and chicken into four portions.

Nutrients per serving:
Calories: 294, **Calories from Fat:** 27%, **Total Fat:** 9g, **Saturated Fat:** 1g, **Cholesterol:** 65mg, **Sodium:** 217mg, **Carbohydrate:** 22g, **Fiber:** 8g, **Protein:** 31g

Dietary Exchange: 1 Starch, 1 Vegetable, 3 Meat

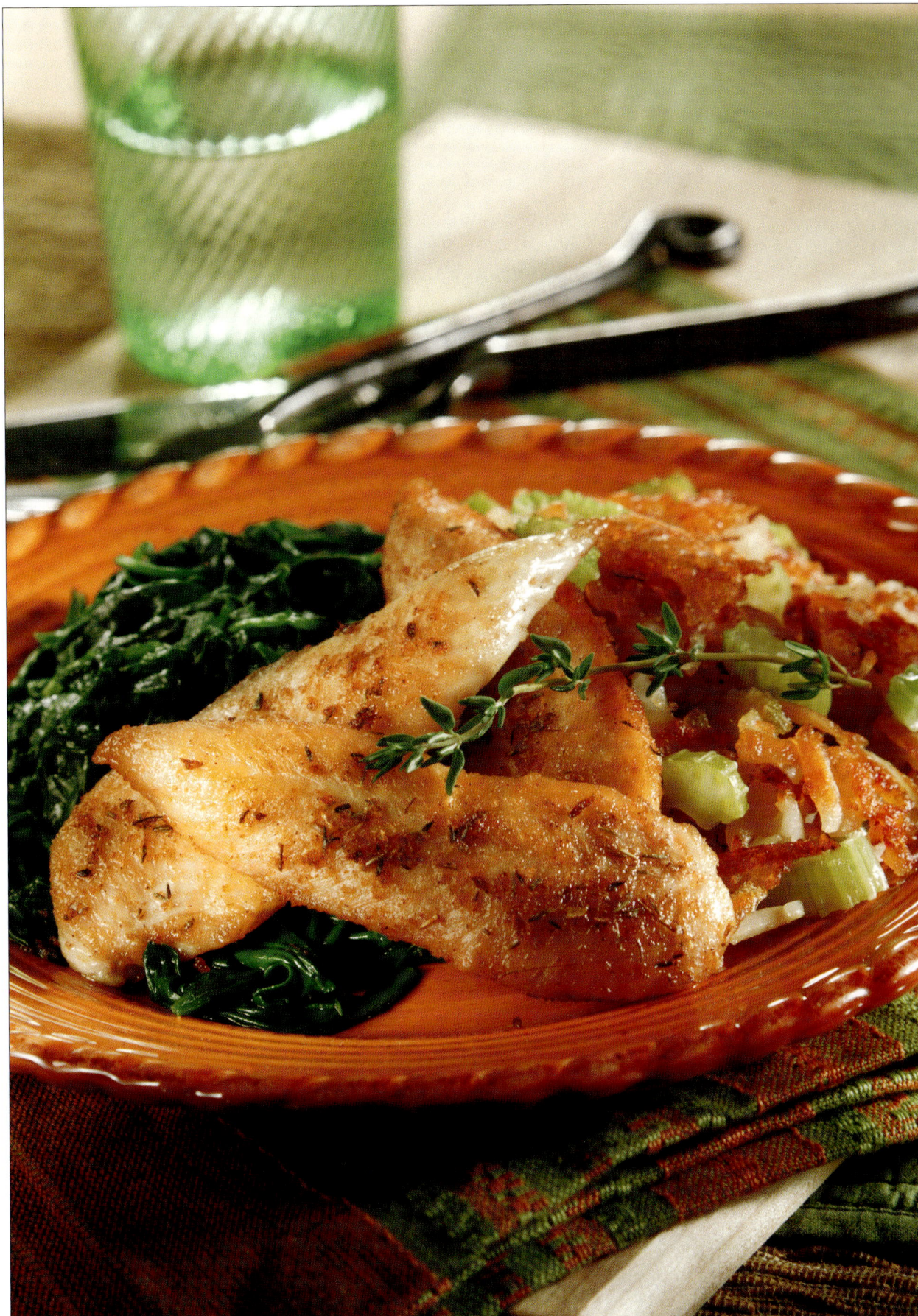

Chicken with Spinach and Celery-Potato Hash

Mushroom Pasta Scampi

Makes 4 servings

- 8 ounces uncooked linguine
- 2 tablespoons olive oil
- 1 pound fresh white mushrooms, sliced
- 1 tablespoon chopped garlic
- 1 pound frozen raw peeled and deveined large shrimp, thawed*
- 10 ounces fresh spinach, trimmed and torn into pieces (about 7 cups)
- ¼ cup grated Parmesan cheese
- ¼ teaspoon crushed red pepper

To quickly thaw shrimp, place in a colander under cold running water for about 8 minutes; drain thoroughly.

Cook linguine according to package directions. Drain, reserving ½ cup pasta water; set aside. Meanwhile, heat olive oil in large skillet. Add mushrooms and garlic; cook and stir about 5 minutes or until tender and mushroom liquid is almost evaporated. Add shrimp; cover and cook about 5 minutes or until shrimp is almost cooked through. Stir in spinach and reserved ½ cup pasta water, if desired. Cover and cook about 1 minute or until spinach is wilted. Place pasta in serving bowl; stir in mushroom and shrimp mixtures, Parmesan cheese and red pepper. Toss to combine. Season with salt, if desired.

Favorite recipe from **Mushroom Information Center**

Preparation and Cooking Time: about 15 minutes

Nutrients per serving: 1½ cups Scampi (without salt seasoning)
Calories: 415, **Calories from Fat:** 29%, **Total Fat:** 13g,
Saturated Fat: 3g, **Cholesterol:** 240mg, **Sodium:** 370mg,
Carbohydrate: 38g, **Fiber:** 9g, **Protein:** 37g

Dietary Exchange: 2 Starch, 1 Vegetable, 4 Meat, ½ Fat

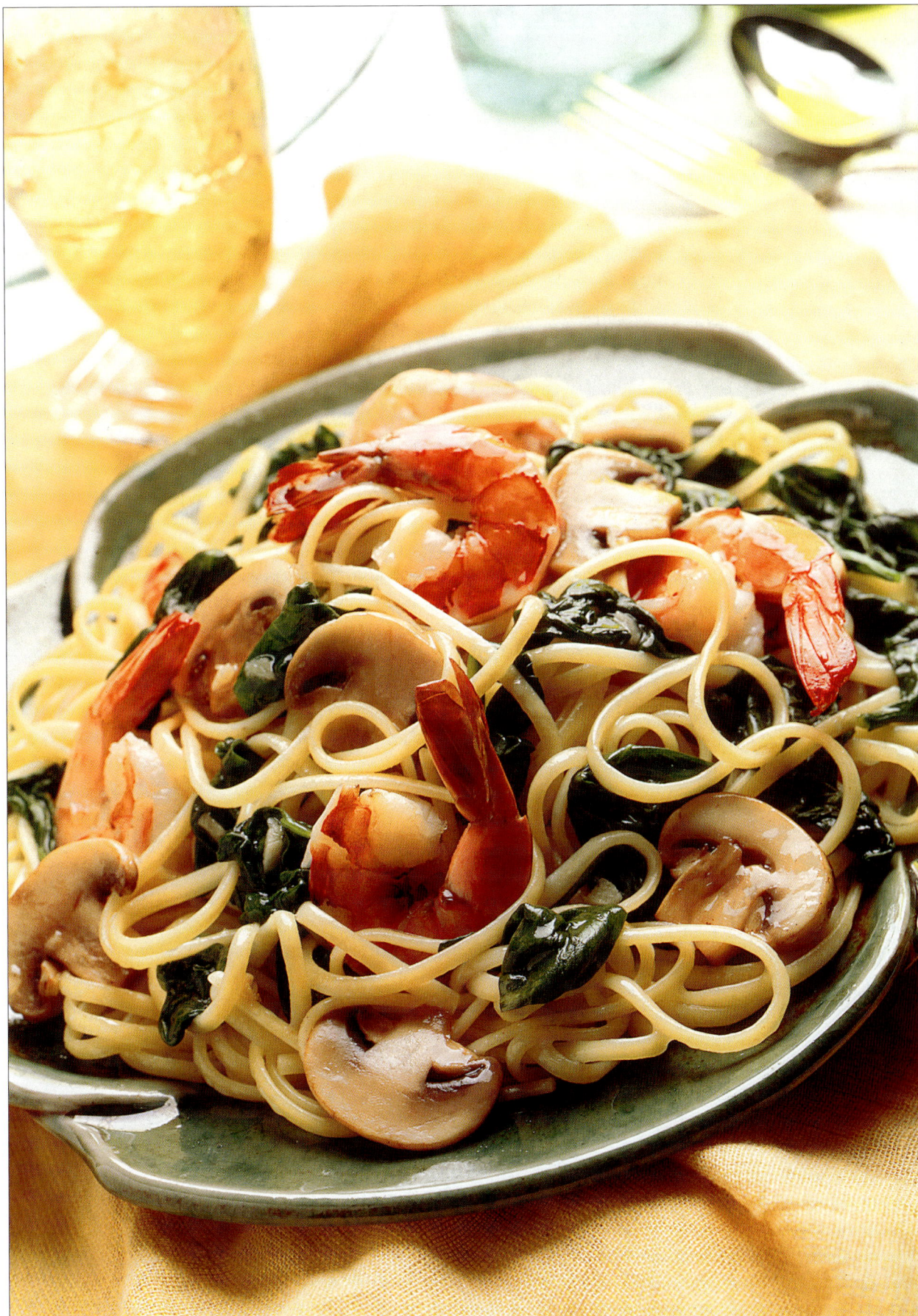

Mushroom Pasta Scampi

Thai-Style Pork Kabobs

Makes 4 servings

- ⅓ cup reduced-sodium soy sauce
- 2 tablespoons water
- 2 tablespoons fresh lime juice
- 2 teaspoons hot chili oil*
- 2 cloves garlic, minced
- 1 teaspoon minced fresh ginger
- 12 ounces well-trimmed pork tenderloin
- 1 red or yellow bell pepper, cut into ½-inch pieces
- 1 red or sweet onion, cut into ½-inch chunks
- 2 cups hot cooked rice

If hot chili oil is not available, combine 2 teaspoons vegetable oil and ½ teaspoon red pepper flakes in small microwavable cup. Microwave at HIGH 30 to 45 seconds. Let stand 5 minutes to allow flavor to develop.

1. Combine soy sauce, water, lime juice, chili oil, garlic and ginger in medium bowl. Reserve ⅓ cup mixture for dipping sauce; set aside.

2. Cut pork tenderloin lengthwise in half; cut crosswise into 4-inch-thick slices. Cut slices into ½-inch strips. Add to bowl with soy sauce mixture; toss to coat. Cover; refrigerate at least 30 minutes or up to 2 hours, turning once.

3. Spray grid with nonstick cooking spray to prevent sticking. Prepare grill for direct grilling.

4. Remove pork from marinade; discard marinade. Alternately weave pork strips and thread bell pepper and onion chunks onto eight 8- to 10-inch metal skewers.

5. Grill, covered, over medium-hot coals 6 to 8 minutes or until pork is barely pink in center, turning halfway through grilling time. Serve with rice and reserved dipping sauce.

Nutrients per serving: 2 Kabobs with ½ cup rice and about 1 tablespoon plus 1 teaspoon dipping sauce
Calories: 248, **Calories from Fat:** 16%, **Total Fat:** 4g,
Saturated Fat: 1g, **Cholesterol:** 49mg, **Sodium:** 271mg,
Carbohydrate: 30g, **Fiber:** 2g, **Protein:** 22g

Dietary Exchange: 1½ Starch, 1 Vegetable, 2 Meat

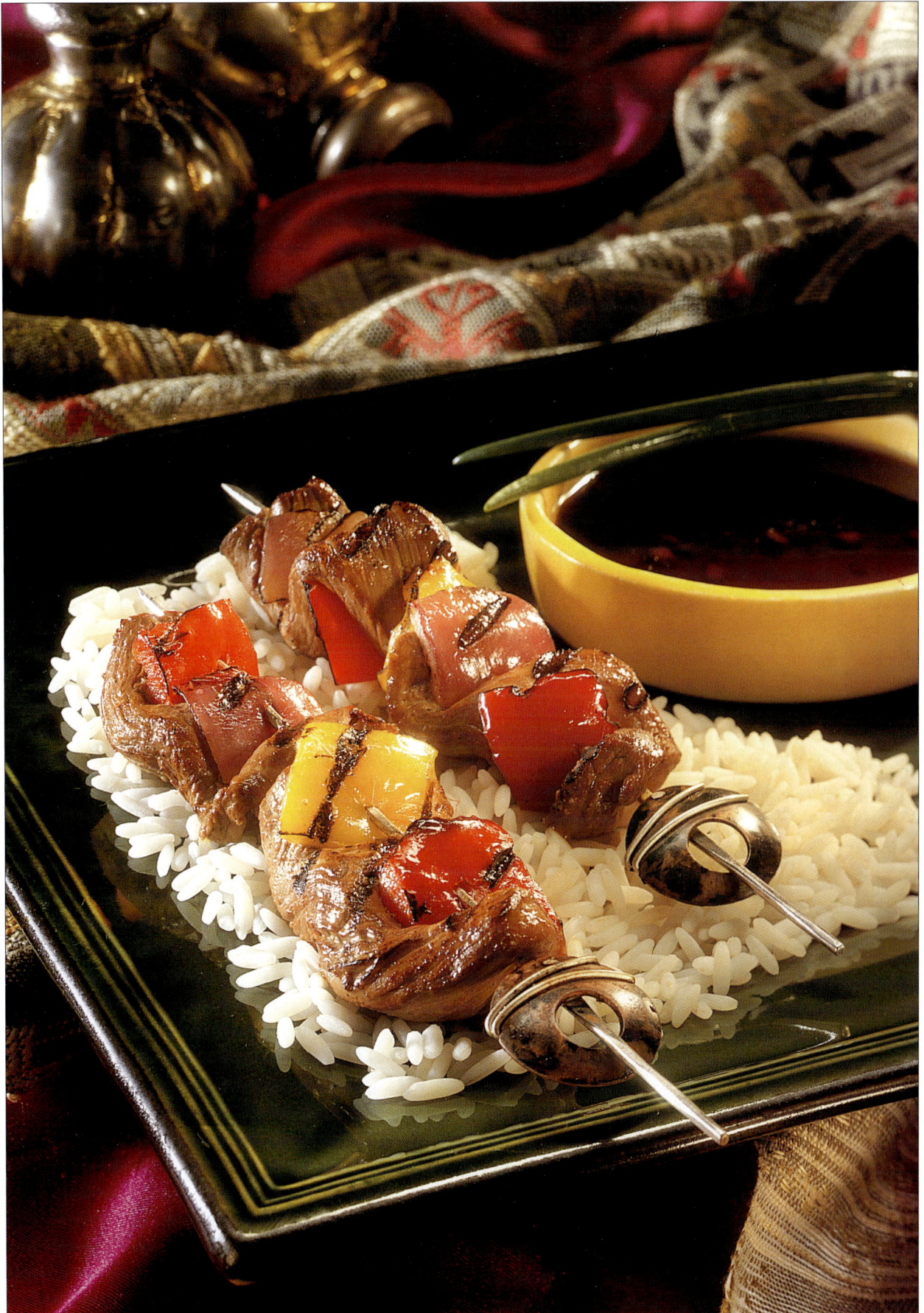

Thai-Style Pork Kabobs

Italian Crouton Salad

Makes 6 servings

  6 **ounces French or Italian bread**
  ¼ **cup plain nonfat yogurt**
  ¼ **cup red wine vinegar**
  4 **teaspoons olive oil**
  1 **tablespoon water**
  3 **cloves garlic, minced**
  6 **medium (about 12 ounces) plum tomatoes**
  ½ **medium red onion, thinly sliced**
  3 **tablespoons slivered fresh basil leaves**
  2 **tablespoons finely chopped fresh parsley**
 12 **leaves red leaf lettuce** *or* **4 cups prepared Italian salad mix**
  2 **tablespoons grated Parmesan cheese**

1. Preheat broiler. To prepare croutons, cut bread into ¾-inch cubes. Place in single layer on baking sheet. Broil, 4 inches from heat, 3 minutes or until bread is golden, stirring every 30 seconds to 1 minute. Remove from baking sheet; place in large bowl.

2. Whisk together yogurt, vinegar, oil, water and garlic in small bowl until blended; set aside. Core tomatoes; cut into ¼-inch-wide slices. Add to croutons along with onion, basil and parsley; stir until blended. Pour yogurt mixture over crouton mixture; toss to coat. Cover; refrigerate 30 minutes or up to 1 day. (Croutons will be more tender the following day.)

3. To serve, place lettuce on plates. Spoon crouton mixture over lettuce. Sprinkle with Parmesan cheese.

Nutrients per serving:
Calories: 160, **Calories from Fat:** 28%, **Total Fat:** 5g,
Saturated Fat: 1g, **Cholesterol:** 2mg, **Sodium:** 234mg,
Carbohydrate: 25g, **Fiber:** 2g, **Protein:** 6g

Dietary Exchange: 1 Starch, 1½ Vegetable, 1 Fat

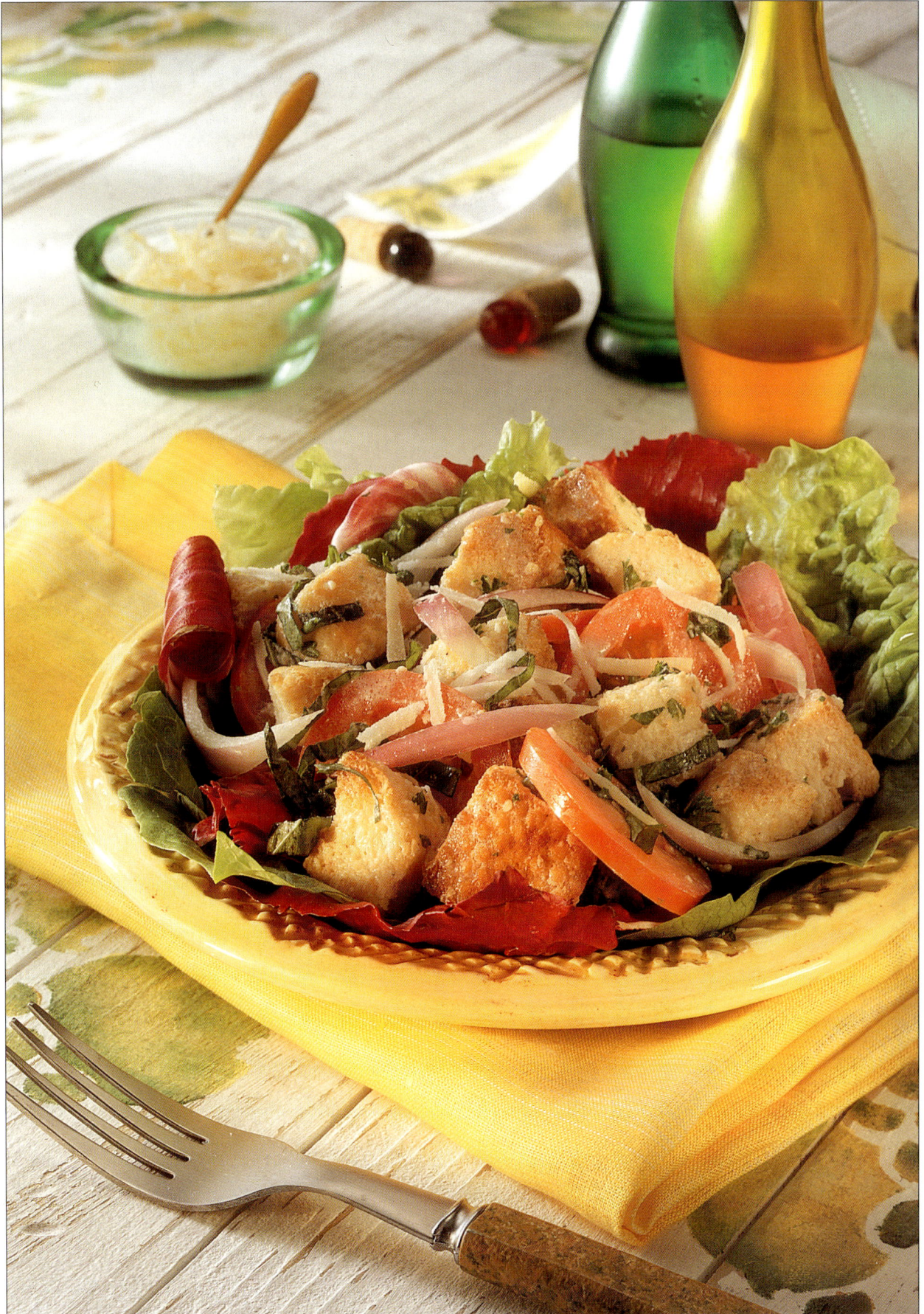

Italian Crouton Salad

cooking for two

Teriyaki Salmon with Asian Slaw

Makes 2 servings

  4 tablespoons light teriyaki sauce, divided
  2 (5- to 6-ounce) boneless salmon fillets with skin (1 inch thick)
2½ cups packaged coleslaw mix
  1 cup fresh or frozen pea pods cut lengthwise into thin strips
  ½ cup thinly sliced radishes
  2 tablespoons orange marmalade
  1 teaspoon dark sesame oil

1. Preheat broiler or prepare grill for direct cooking. Spoon 2 tablespoons teriyaki sauce over meaty sides of salmon. Let stand while preparing vegetable mixture.

2. Combine cole slaw mix, pea pods and radishes in large bowl. Combine remaining 2 tablespoons teriyaki sauce, marmalade and sesame oil in small bowl. Add to coleslaw mixture; toss well.

3. Broil salmon 4 to 5 inches from heat source or grill, flesh side down, over medium coals without turning 6 to 10 minutes until center is opaque.

4. Transfer coleslaw mixture to serving plates; top with salmon.

Nutrients per serving:
Calories: 354, **Calories from Fat:** 28%, **Total Fat:** 11g,
Saturated Fat: 2g, **Cholesterol:** 75mg, **Sodium:** 730mg,
Carbohydrate: 32g, **Fiber:** 5g, **Protein:** 32g

Dietary Exchange: 1 Starch, 2 Vegetable, 4 Meat

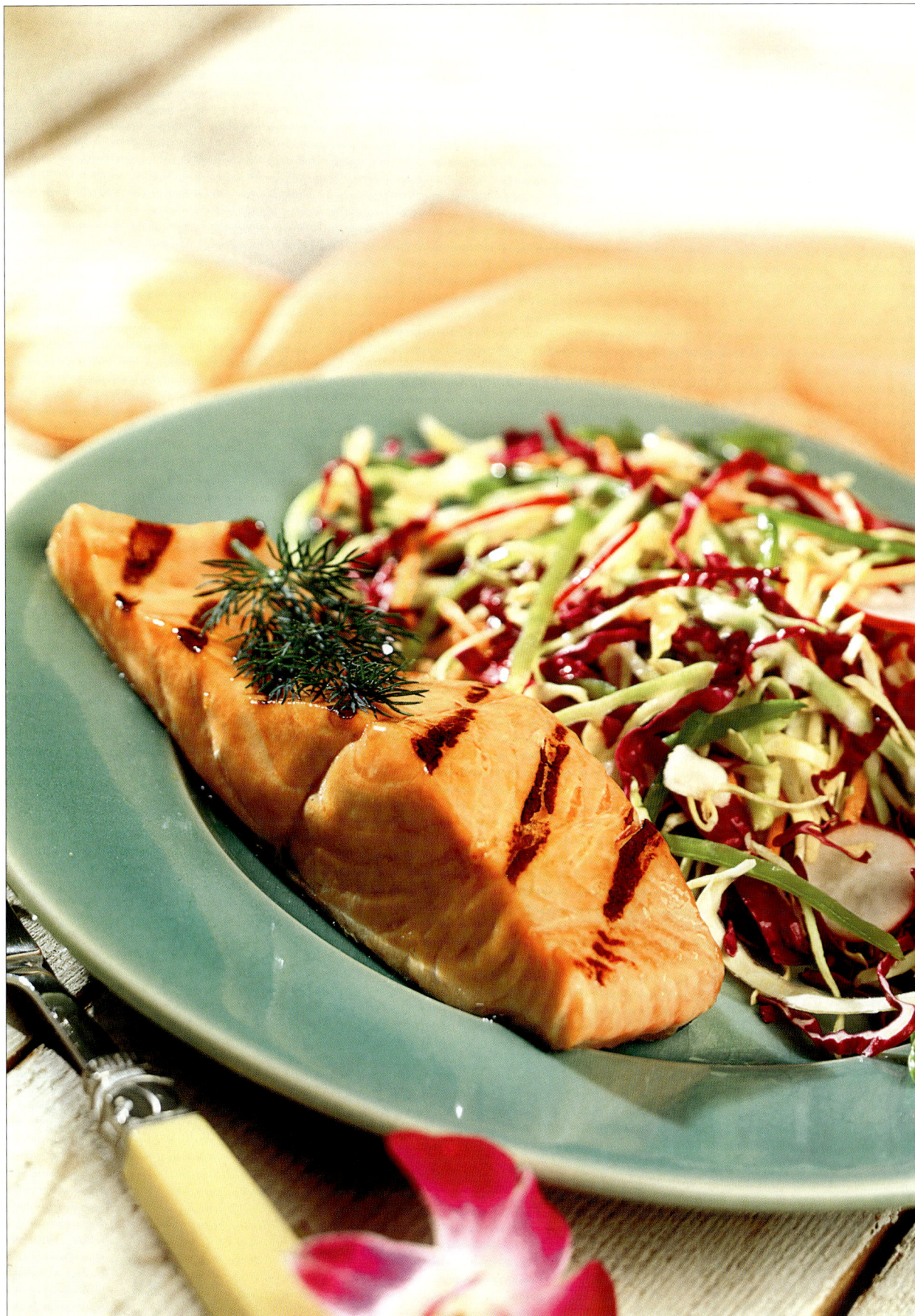

Teriyaki Salmon with Asian Slaw

Sassy Chicken & Peppers

Makes 2 servings

- 2 teaspoons Mexican seasoning*
- 2 (4-ounce) boneless skinless chicken breasts
- 2 teaspoons canola oil
- 1 small red onion, sliced
- ½ red bell pepper, cut into long, thin strips
- ½ yellow or green bell pepper, cut into long, thin strips
- ¼ cup chunky salsa or chipotle salsa
- 1 tablespoon lime juice
     Lime wedges (optional)

*If Mexican seasoning is not available, substitute 1 teaspoon chili powder, ½ teaspoon ground cumin, ½ teaspoon salt and ⅛ teaspoon ground red pepper.

1. Sprinkle seasoning over both sides of chicken.

2. Heat oil in large nonstick skillet over medium heat. Add onion; cook 3 minutes, stirring occasionally.

3. Add bell pepper strips; cook 3 minutes, stirring occasionally.

4. Push vegetables to edges of skillet; add chicken to skillet. Cook 5 minutes; turn. Stir salsa and lime juice into vegetables. Continue to cook 4 minutes or until chicken is no longer pink in the center and vegetables are tender.

5. Transfer chicken to serving plates; top with vegetable mixture and garnish with lime wedges, if desired.

Nutrients per serving:
Calories: 224, **Calories from Fat:** 31%, **Total Fat:** 8g,
Saturated Fat: 1g, **Cholesterol:** 69mg, **Sodium:** 813mg,
Carbohydrate: 11g, **Fiber:** 3g, **Protein:** 27g

Dietary Exchange: 2 Vegetable, 3 Meat

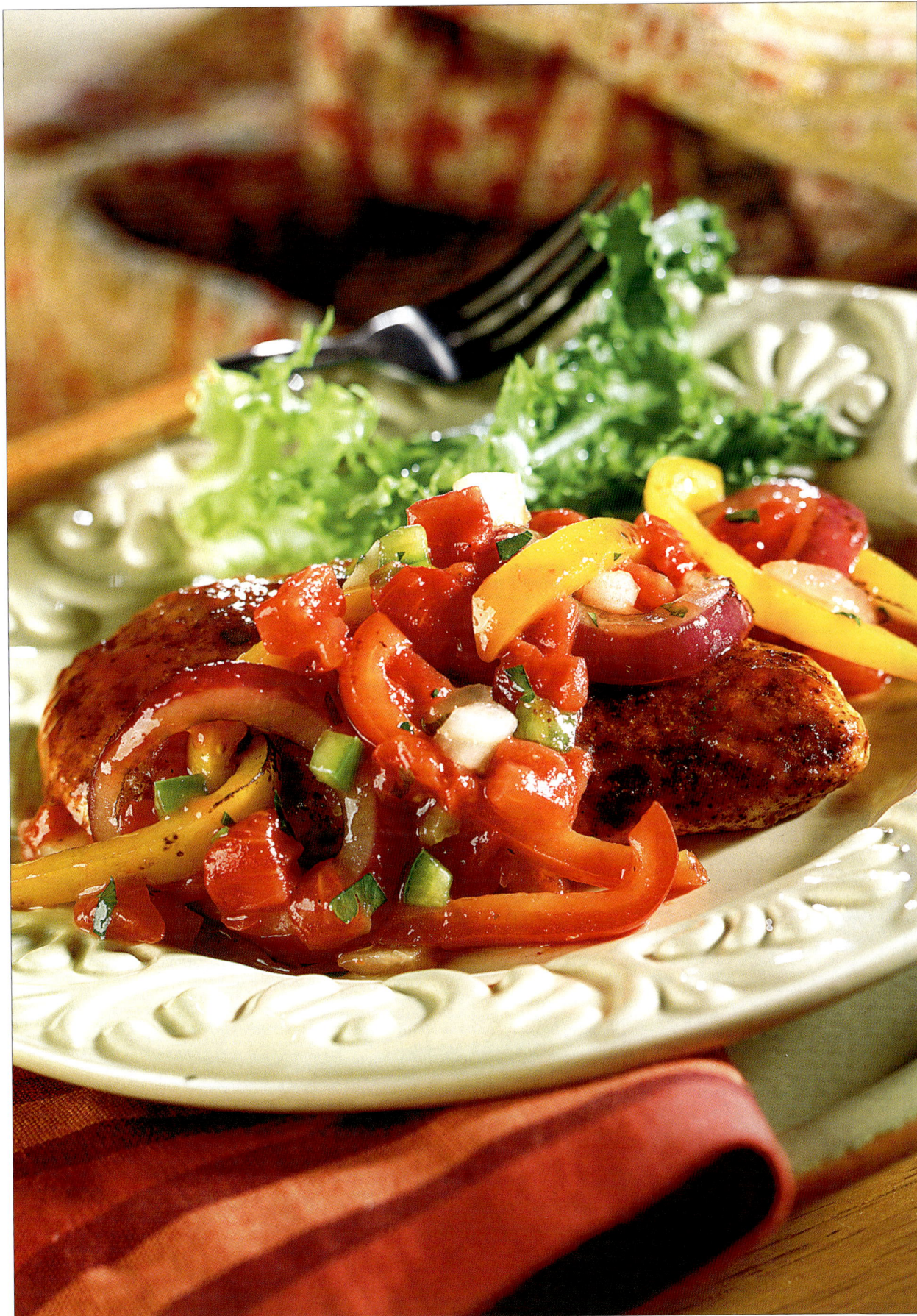

Sassy Chicken & Peppers

Chili Beef & Red Pepper Fajitas with Chipotle Salsa

Makes 2 servings

- 6 ounces boneless beef top sirloin steak, thinly sliced
- ½ lime
- 1½ teaspoons chili powder
- ½ teaspoon ground cumin
- ½ cup diced plum tomatoes
- ¼ cup mild picante sauce
- ½ canned chipotle chili pepper in adobo sauce
  Nonstick cooking spray
- ½ cup sliced onion
- ½ red bell pepper, cut into thin strips
- 2 (10-inch) fat-free flour tortillas, warmed
- ¼ cup fat-free sour cream
- 2 tablespoons chopped fresh cilantro leaves (optional)

1. Place steak on plate. Squeeze lime juice over steak; sprinkle with chili powder and cumin. Coat well; let stand 10 minutes.

2. Meanwhile, to prepare salsa, combine tomatoes and picante sauce in small bowl. Place chipotle on small plate. Using fork, mash completely. Stir mashed chipotle into tomato mixture.

3. Coat 12-inch skillet with cooking spray. Heat over high heat until hot. Add onion and bell pepper; cook and stir 3 minutes or until edges begin to blacken. Remove from skillet. Lightly spray skillet with cooking spray. Add beef; stir-fry 1 minute. Return onion and bell pepper to skillet; cook 1 minute longer.

4. Place ½ the beef mixture in center of each tortilla; fold sides over filling. Top each fajita with ¼ cup salsa, 2 tablespoons sour cream and cilantro, if desired.

Note: For a less spicy salsa, use less chipotle chili or eliminate it completely.

Nutrients per serving: 1 Fajita with ¼ cup Salsa and 2 tablespoons fat-free sour cream (without garnish)
Calories: 245, **Calories from Fat:** 16%, **Total Fat:** 4g, **Saturated Fat:** 2g, **Cholesterol:** 45mg, **Sodium:** 530mg, **Carbohydrate:** 31g, **Fiber:** 9g, **Protein:** 21g

Dietary Exchange: 1½ Starch, 1 Vegetable, 2 Meat

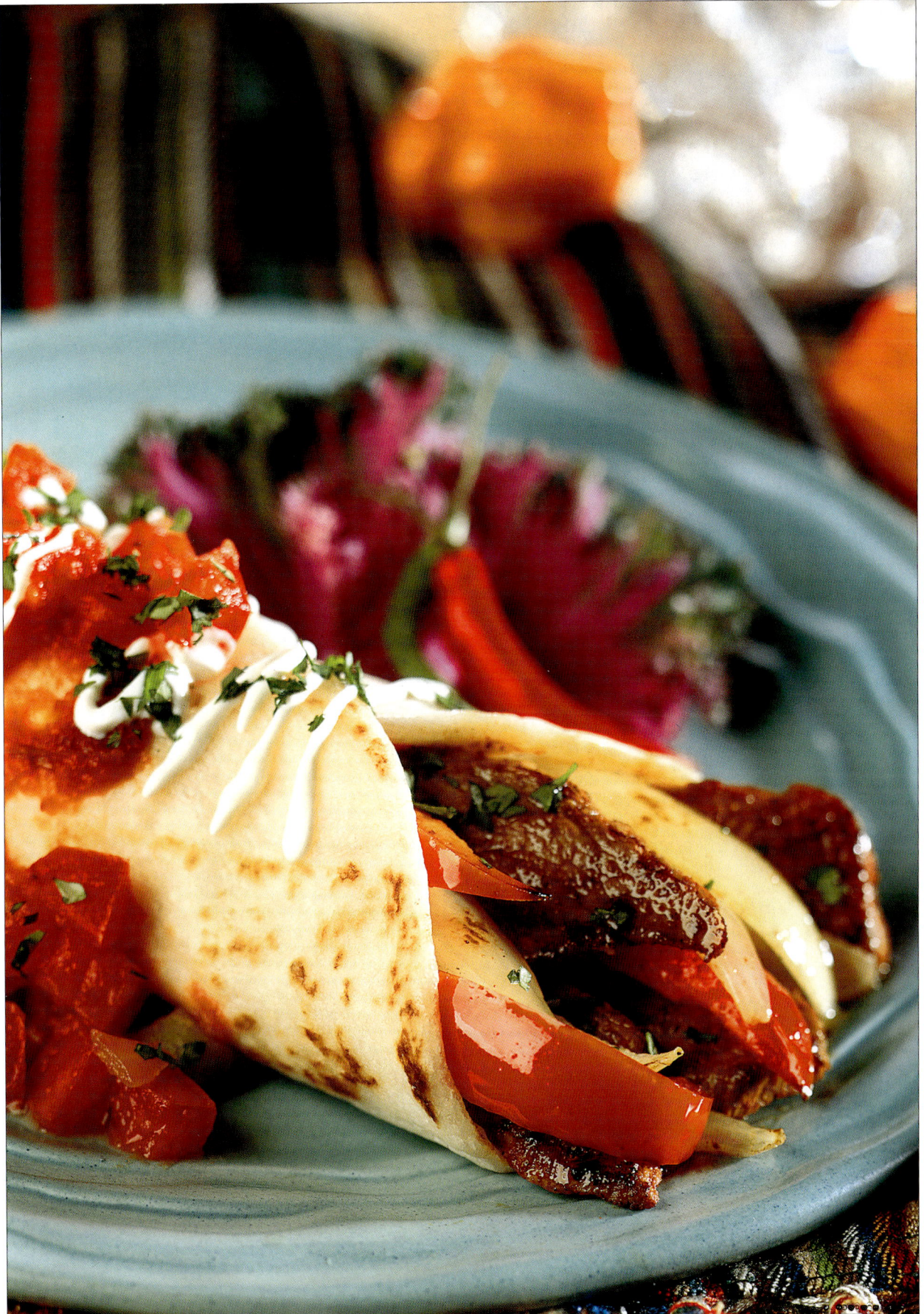

Chili Beef & Red Pepper Fajita with Chipotle Salsa

Lemon Chicken Stir-Fry

Makes 2 servings

- ½ **cup vegetable broth or water**
- 4 **tablespoons lemon juice**
- 2 **teaspoons cornstarch**
- 2 **teaspoons apple juice or dry sherry**
- 2 **teaspoons soy sauce**
- 1 **teaspoon chili sauce**
- 1 **chicken-flavored bouillon cube**
- 1 **tablespoon oil, divided**
- 2 **boneless, skinless chicken breasts (8 ounces), cut into strips**
- 2 **cloves garlic, crushed**
- 1 **onion, thinly sliced**
- 1 **carrot, thinly sliced**
- ½ **cup celery, thinly sliced**
- ½ **cup zucchini, sliced**
- 8 **snow peas**
- ¼ **cup sliced green or red pepper**
- 2 **tablespoons EQUAL® SPOONFUL***

*May substitute 3 packets Equal® sweetener or 1 teaspoon Equal® for Recipes.

- For lemon sauce, blend vegetable broth, lemon juice, cornstarch, apple juice, soy sauce, chili sauce and chicken-flavored bouillon cube in small bowl until smooth. Set aside.

- Heat half of oil in wok or heavy frying pan. Cook and stir chicken and garlic until lightly browned. Set aside.

- Add remaining oil to pan. Sauté vegetables about 3 minutes until heated through.

- Return chicken to pan; add lemon sauce and cook until sauce is slightly thickened and bubbling. Stir in Equal®; cook and stir until sauce boils and thickens. Serve over rice, if desired.

Nutrients per serving:
Calories: 287, **Calories from Fat:** 25%, **Total Fat:** 9g,
Cholesterol: 69mg, **Sodium:** 1,015mg, **Carbohydrate:** 22g,
Protein: 30g

Dietary Exchange: 4 Vegetable, 3 Meat

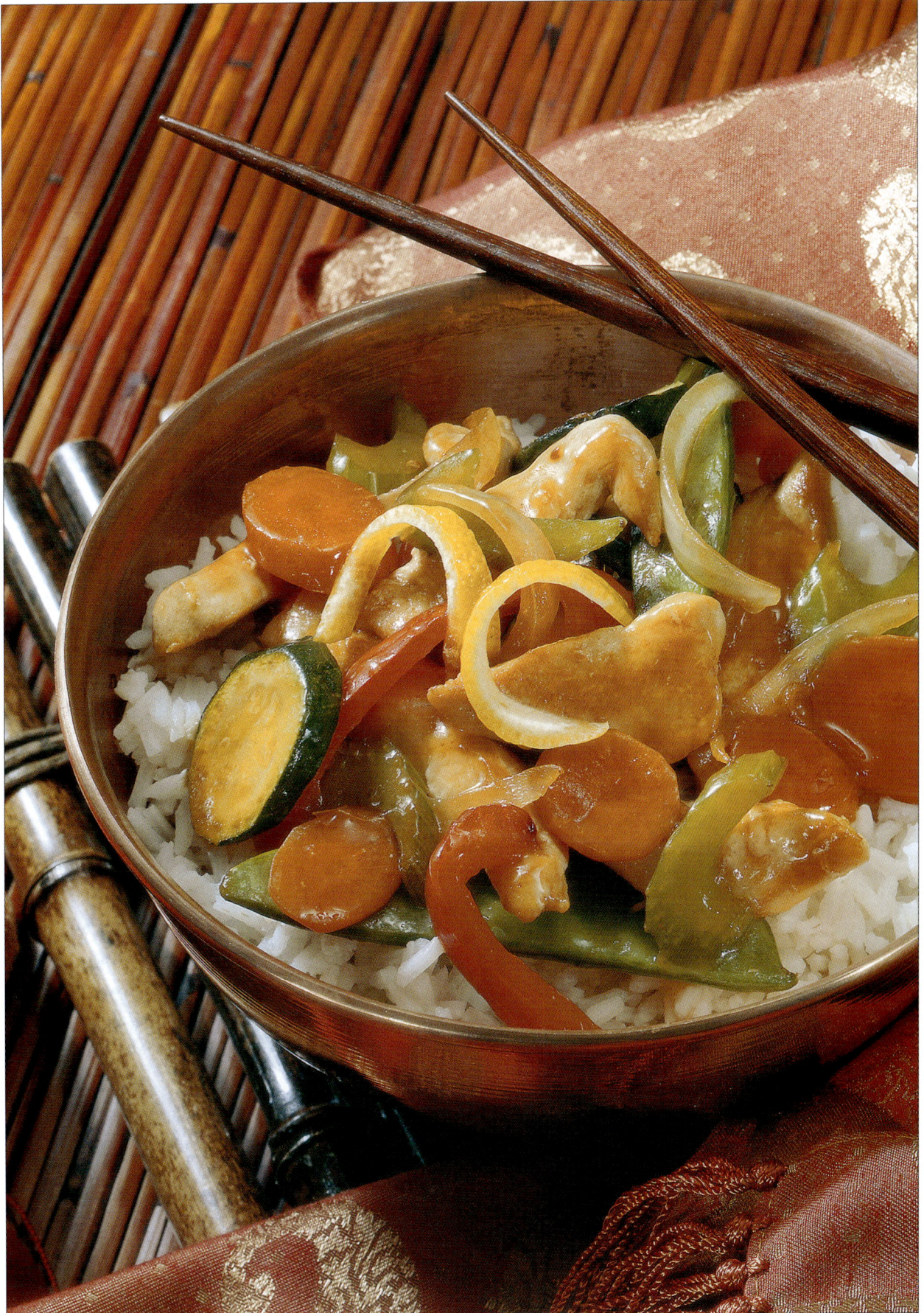

Lemon Chicken Stir-Fry

Apple-Cherry Glazed Pork Chops

Makes 2 servings

- 2 boneless pork loin chops (3 ounces each)
- ¼ to ½ teaspoon dried thyme leaves
- ⅛ teaspoon salt
- ⅛ teaspoon black pepper
- Nonstick olive oil cooking spray
- ⅔ cup unsweetened apple juice
- ½ small apple, peeled and sliced
- 2 tablespoons sliced green onion
- 2 tablespoons dried tart cherries
- 1 tablespoon water
- 1 teaspoon cornstarch

1. Trim fat from pork chops. Stir together thyme, salt and pepper. Rub on both sides of pork chops. Spray large skillet with cooking spray. Add pork chops. Cook over medium heat 3 to 5 minutes or until barely pink in center, turning once. Remove chops from skillet; keep warm.

2. Add apple juice, apple slices, green onion and cherries to same skillet. Simmer, uncovered, 2 to 3 minutes or until apple and onions are tender. Mix water and cornstarch in small bowl. Add to mixture in skillet; cook and stir until boiling. Serve over pork chops.

Nutrients per serving:
Calories: 243, **Calories from Fat:** 31%, **Total Fat:** 8g, **Saturated Fat:** 3g, **Cholesterol:** 40mg, **Sodium:** 191mg, **Carbohydrate:** 23g, **Fiber:** 1g, **Protein:** 19g

Dietary Exchange: 1½ Fruit, 2 Meat, 1 Fat

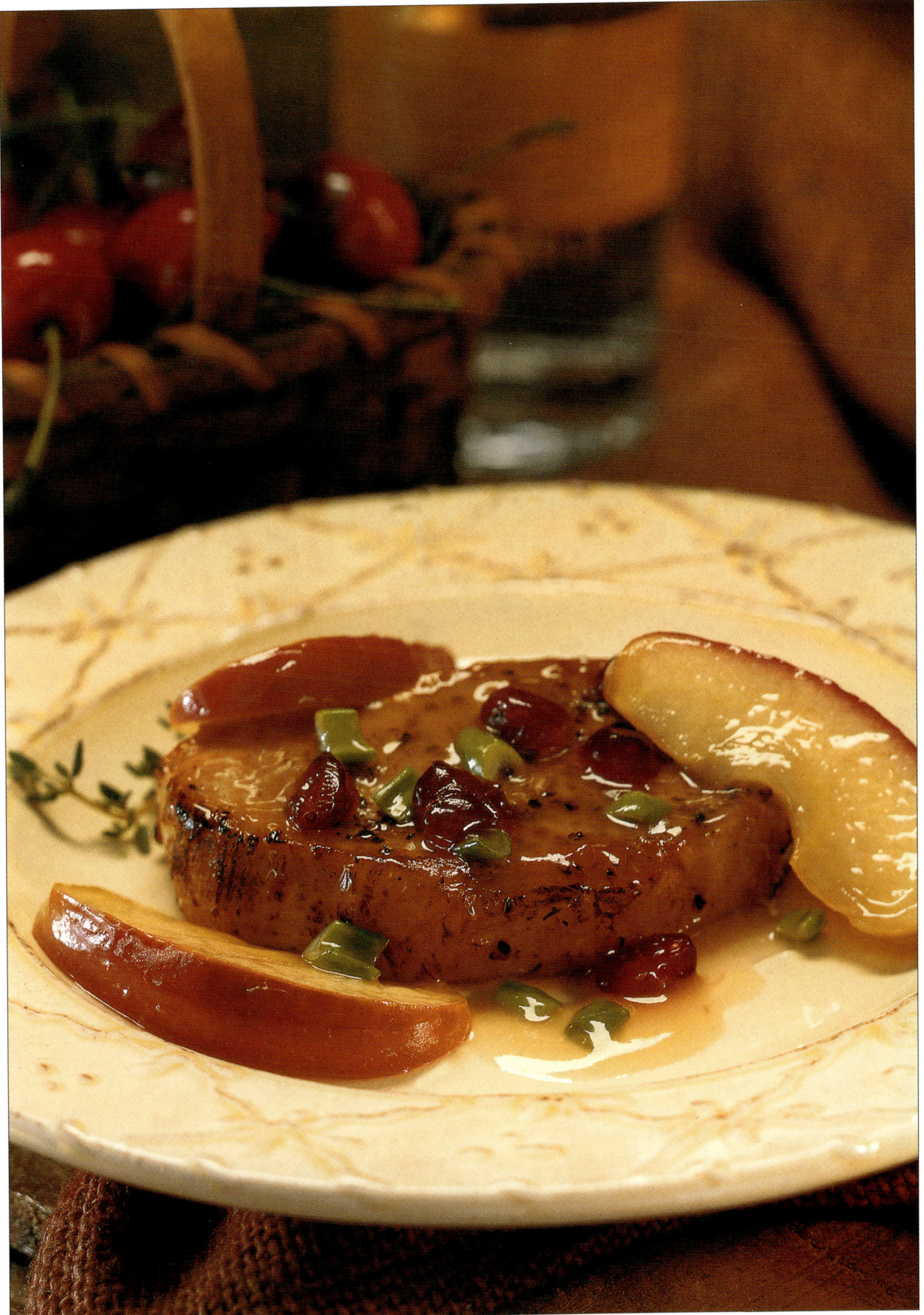

Apple-Cherry Glazed Pork Chop

Grilled Salmon Salad with Orange-Basil Vinaigrette

Makes 2 servings

- ¼ cup frozen orange juice concentrate, thawed
- 1 tablespoon plus 1½ teaspoons white wine vinegar or cider vinegar
- 1 tablespoon chopped basil *or* 1 teaspoon dried basil leaves
- 1½ teaspoons olive oil
- 1 (8-ounce) salmon fillet (about 1 inch thick)
- 4 cups torn mixed greens
- ¾ cup sliced strawberries
- 10 to 12 thin cucumber slices, cut into halves
- ⅛ teaspoon coarsely ground black pepper

1. Whisk together juice concentrate, vinegar, basil and olive oil. Set aside 2 tablespoons juice concentrate mixture. Reserve remaining mixture to use as salad dressing.

2. Prepare grill for direct grilling. Grill salmon, skin side down, over medium coals 5 minutes. Turn and grill 5 minutes or until fish flakes easily with fork, brushing frequently with 2 tablespoons juice concentrate mixture. Cool slightly.

3. Toss greens, strawberries and cucumber slices in large bowl. Divide evenly between two plates.

4. Remove skin from salmon. Break salmon into chunks. Arrange salmon on salad. Drizzle with reserved juice concentrate mixture. Sprinkle with pepper.

Nutrients per serving:
Calories: 283, **Calories from Fat:** 35%, **Total Fat:** 11g,
Saturated Fat: 2g, **Cholesterol:** 60mg, **Sodium:** 70mg,
Carbohydrate: 23g, **Fiber:** 3g, **Protein:** 24g

Dietary Exchange: 1½ Fruit, 3 Meat, ½ Fat

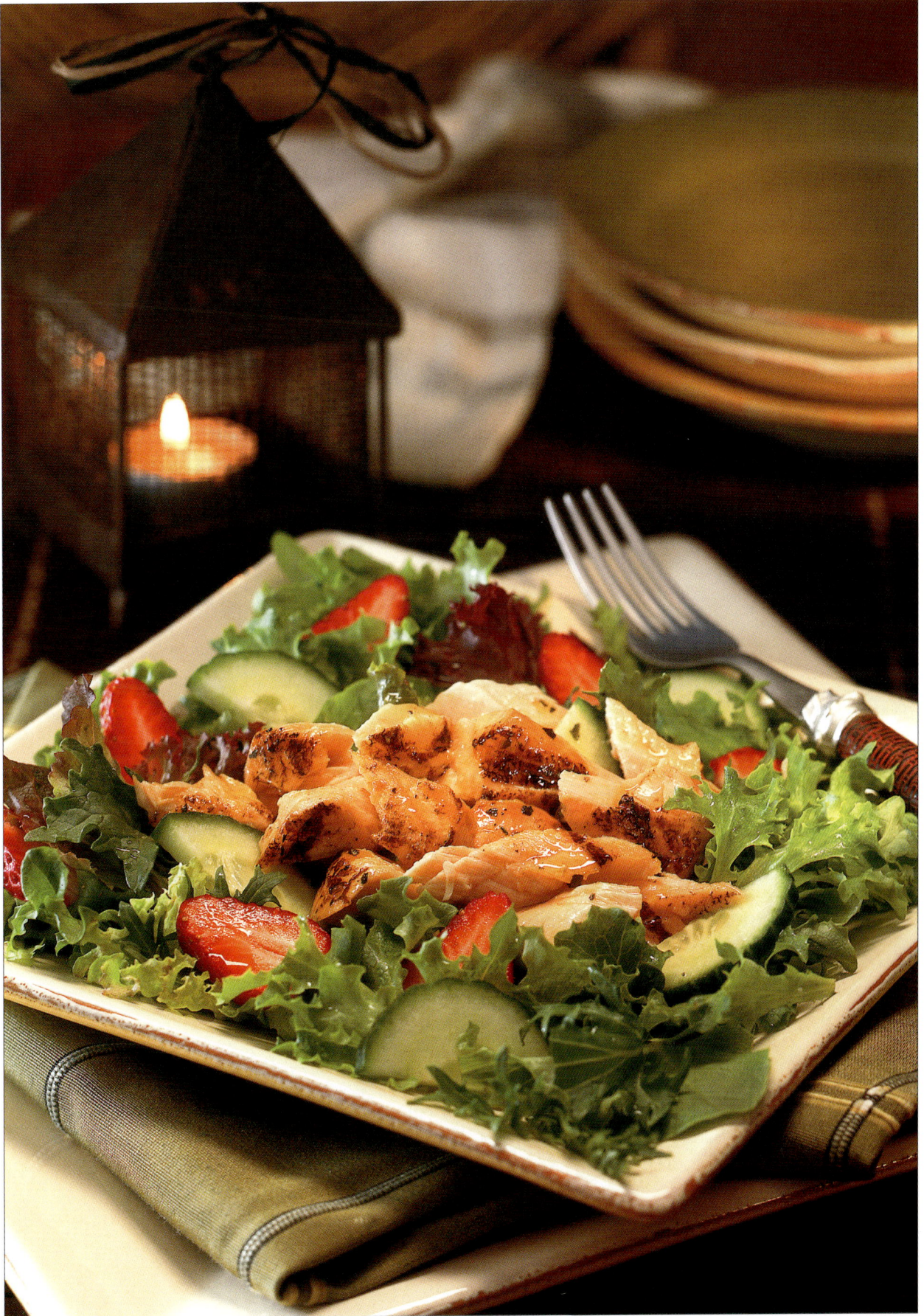

Grilled Salmon Salad with Orange-Basil Vinaigrette

Spinach & Turkey Skillet

Makes 2 servings

- 6 ounces turkey breast tenderloin
- ⅛ teaspoon salt
- 2 teaspoons olive oil
- ¼ cup chopped onion
- 2 cloves garlic, minced
- ⅓ cup uncooked rice
- ¾ teaspoon dried Italian seasoning
- ¼ teaspoon black pepper
- 1 cup fat-free reduced-sodium chicken broth, divided
- 2 cups torn fresh spinach leaves
- ⅔ cup diced plum tomatoes
- 3 tablespoons freshly grated Parmesan cheese

1. Cut turkey tenderloins into bite-size pieces; sprinkle with salt.

2. Heat oil in medium skillet over medium-high heat. Add turkey pieces; cook and stir until lightly browned. Remove from skillet. Reduce heat to low. Add onion and garlic; cook and stir until tender. Return turkey to skillet. Stir in rice, Italian seasoning and pepper.

3. Reserve 2 tablespoons chicken broth. Stir remaining broth into mixture in skillet. Bring to a boil. Reduce heat; simmer, covered, 14 minutes. Stir in spinach and reserved broth. Cover; cook 2 to 3 minutes or until liquid is absorbed and spinach is wilted. Stir in tomatoes; heat through. Serve with Parmesan cheese.

Nutrients per serving: ½ of total recipe
Calories: 316, **Calories from Fat:** 26%, **Total Fat:** 9g,
Saturated Fat: 3g, **Cholesterol:** 39mg, **Sodium:** 309mg,
Carbohydrate: 33g, **Fiber:** 3g, **Protein:** 25g

Dietary Exchange: 2 Starch, 3 Meat

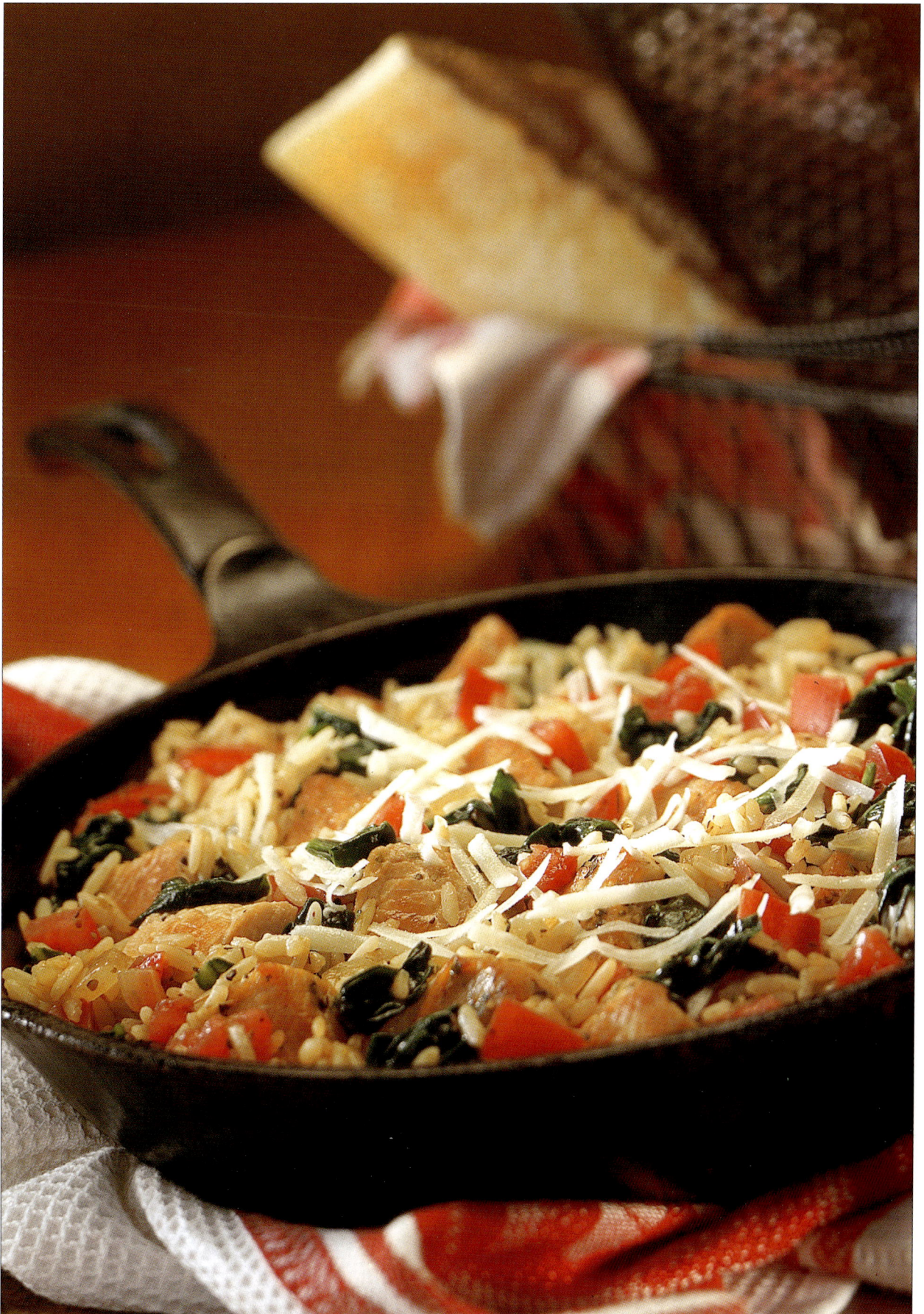

Spinach & Turkey Skillet

cooking for kids

Finger Licking Chicken Salad

Makes 1 serving

- ½ cup purchased carved roasted skinless chicken breast, cubed
- ½ rib celery, cut into 1-inch pieces
- ¼ cup drained mandarin orange segments
- ¼ cup red seedless grapes
- 2 tablespoons fat-free, sugar-free lemon yogurt
- 1 tablespoon reduced-fat mayonnaise
- ¼ teaspoon reduced-sodium soy sauce
- ⅛ teaspoon pumpkin pie spice or cinnamon

1. Toss chicken, celery, oranges and grapes in covered plastic container.

2. For dipping sauce, combine yogurt, mayonnaise, soy sauce and pumpkin pie spice in small covered plastic container.

3. Pack chicken mixture and dipping sauce in insulated bag with ice pack. To serve, dip chicken mixture into dipping sauce.

Variation: Alternately thread the chicken, celery, oranges and grapes on wooden skewers.

Nutrients per serving: 1 Salad
Calories: 207, **Calories from Fat:** 25%, **Total Fat:** 6g,
Saturated Fat: 1g, **Cholesterol:** 64mg, **Sodium:** 212mg,
Carbohydrate: 15g, **Fiber:** 1g, **Protein:** 24g

Dietary Exchange: 1 Fruit, 3 Meat

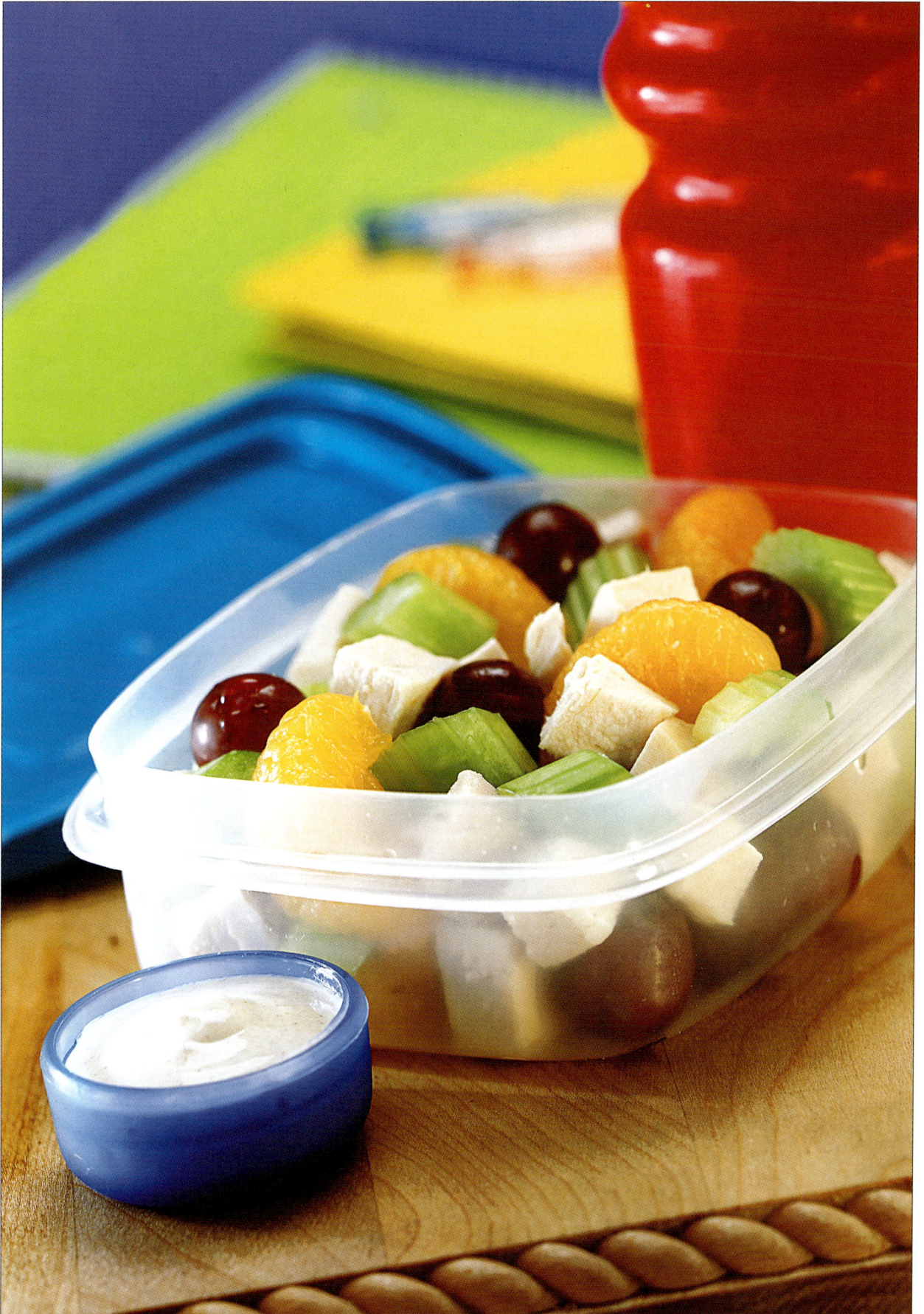

Finger Licking Chicken Salad

Silly Spaghetti Casserole

Makes 6 servings

- 8 **ounces uncooked spaghetti, broken in half**
- ¼ **cup grated Parmesan cheese**
- ¼ **cup cholesterol-free egg substitute**
- ½ **(10-ounce) package frozen cut spinach, thawed**
- ¾ **pound lean ground turkey or 90% lean ground beef**
- ⅓ **cup chopped onion**
- 2 **cups prepared pasta sauce**
- ¾ **cup (3 ounces) shredded part-skim mozzarella cheese**
- 1 **green or yellow bell pepper, cored and seeded**

1. Preheat oven to 350°F. Spray 8-inch square baking dish with nonstick cooking spray.

2. Cook spaghetti according to package directions, omitting salt and oil; drain. Toss with Parmesan cheese and egg substitute. Place in prepared baking dish.

3. Drain spinach in colander, squeezing out excess liquid. Spray large nonstick skillet with cooking spray. Cook turkey and onion in skillet over medium-high heat until meat is lightly browned, stirring to break up meat. Drain off fat. Stir in spinach and spaghetti sauce. Spoon on top of spaghetti mixture.

4. Sprinkle with mozzarella cheese. Use small cookie cutter to cut decorative shapes from bell pepper. Place on top of cheese. Cover with foil. Bake 40 to 45 minutes or until bubbling. Let stand 10 minutes. Cut into squares.

Nutrients per serving: ⅙ of casserole
Calories: 372, **Calories from Fat:** 33%, **Total Fat:** 14g,
Saturated Fat: 6g, **Cholesterol:** 75mg, **Sodium:** 614mg,
Carbohydrate: 39g, **Fiber:** 4g, **Protein:** 23g

Dietary Exchange: 2 Starch, 2 Vegetable, 3 Meat, ½ Fat

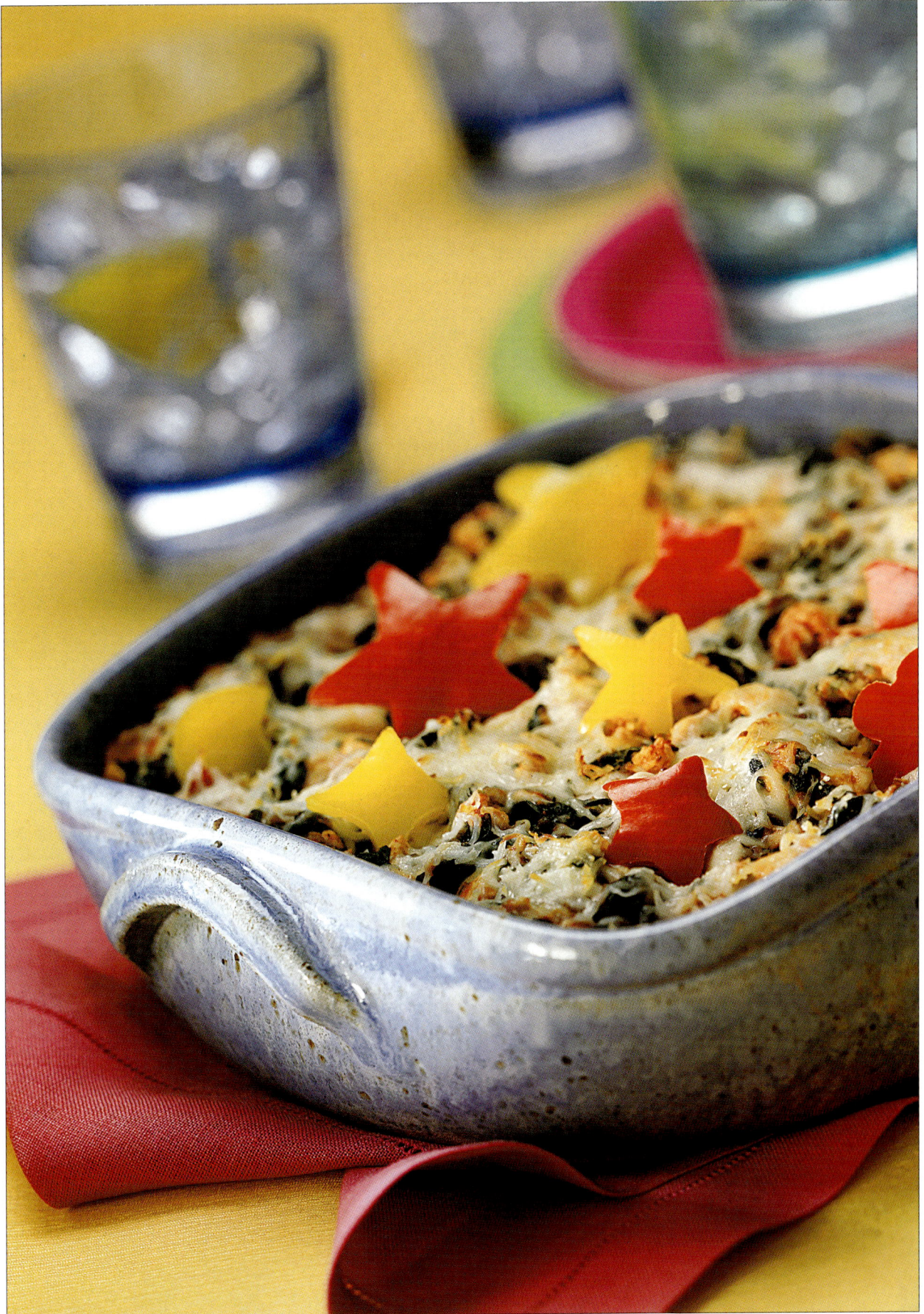

Silly Spaghetti Casserole

Barbecue Flying Saucers with Vegetable Martians

Makes 5 servings

- ½ **teaspoon black pepper***
- 1 **(10-ounce) pork tenderloin***
- ¼ **cup barbecue sauce**
- ½ **teaspoon prepared mustard**
- 1 **(7½-ounce) package (10) refrigerated buttermilk biscuits**
- 1 **egg yolk (optional)**
- 1 **teaspoon water (optional)**
- 3 **to 4 drops food coloring (optional)**
  Vegetable Martians (recipe follows)

*Substitute 10 ounces lean deli roasted pork for pork tenderloin and pepper, if desired.

1. Preheat oven to 425°F. Rub pepper on outside of pork tenderloin. Place pork in shallow roasting pan. Roast 15 to 25 minutes or until meat thermometer inserted into thickest part of meat registers 160°F. Remove from oven; let stand 5 minutes. Shred pork.

2. *Reduce oven temperature to 400°F.* Stir together barbecue sauce and mustard. Toss with shredded pork.

3. Roll each biscuit on lightly floured surface into 4-inch circle. Place one fifth of pork mixture on each of five circles. Moisten edges. Top with remaining biscuit circles. Crimp edges to seal.

4. Stir together egg yolk, water and food coloring to make egg-wash paint, if desired. Using clean paintbrush, paint desired designs on biscuit "flying saucers." Place on baking sheet. Bake 11 to 13 minutes or until golden.

Vegetable Martians: For each Martian, skewer 1 zucchini or cucumber slice, 1 cherry tomato, 2 zucchini or cucumber slices and 1 cherry tomato (for head) on wooden toothpick. Use reduced-fat soft cream cheese or mustard to draw mouth, nose and to attach currants for eyes. Insert 2 chow mein noodles into "head" for antennae. Remove toothpicks before eating.

Nutrients per serving: 1 Flying Saucer plus 1 Vegetable Martian
Calories: 208, **Calories from Fat:** 22%, **Total Fat:** 5g,
Saturated Fat: 1g, **Cholesterol:** 36mg, **Sodium:** 510mg,
Carbohydrate: 26g, **Fiber:** 1g, **Protein:** 15g

Dietary Exchange: 2 Starch, 1 Meat, ½ Fat

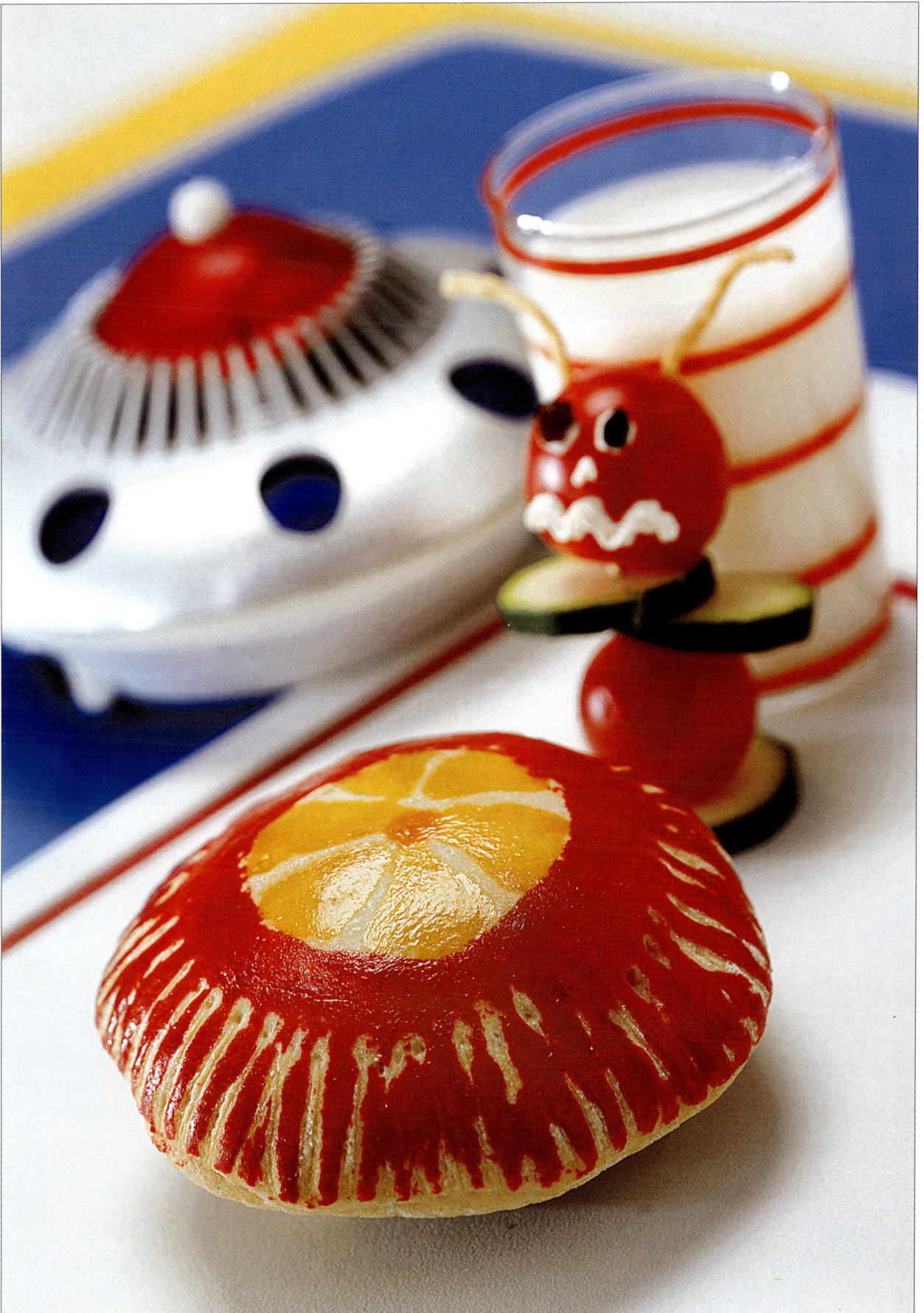

Barbecue Flying Saucer with Vegetable Martian

Chicken Nuggets with Barbecue Dipping Sauce

Makes 8 servings

- 1 **pound boneless skinless chicken breasts**
- ¼ **cup all-purpose flour**
- ¼ **teaspoon salt (optional)**
   Dash black pepper
- 2 **cups crushed reduced-fat baked cheese crackers**
- 1 **teaspoon dried oregano leaves**
- 1 **egg white**
- 1 **tablespoon water**
- 3 **tablespoons barbecue sauce**
- 2 **tablespoons no-sugar-added peach or apricot jam**

1. Preheat oven to 400°F. Cut chicken into 40 (1-inch) pieces.

2. Place flour, salt, if desired, and pepper in resealable plastic food storage bag. Combine cracker crumbs and oregano in shallow bowl. Whisk together egg white and water in small bowl.

3. Place 6 to 8 chicken pieces in bag with flour mixture; seal bag. Shake until chicken is well coated. Remove chicken from bag; shake off excess flour. Dip chicken pieces into egg white mixture, coating all sides. Roll in crumb mixture. Place in shallow baking pan. Repeat with remaining chicken pieces. Bake 10 to 13 minutes or until golden brown.

4. Meanwhile, stir together barbecue sauce and jam in small saucepan. Cook over low heat until hot. (If freezing nuggets, do not prepare dipping sauce at this time.) Serve nuggets with dipping sauce.

Note: To freeze chicken nuggets, wrap 5 cooled nuggets in plastic wrap. Repeat with remaining nuggets. Place packages in freezer bag. Freeze.

Note: To reheat nuggets, preheat oven to 325°F. Place nuggets on ungreased baking sheet. Bake for 13 to 15 minutes or until hot. Or, place 5 nuggets on microwavable plate. Heat on DEFROST (30% power) for 2½ to 3½ minutes or until hot, turning once. For each serving, stir together about 1½ teaspoons barbecue sauce and ½ teaspoon jam in small microwavable dish. Heat on HIGH 10 to 15 seconds or until hot.

Nutrients per serving: 5 Nuggets and scant 2 teaspoons Dipping Sauce
Calories: 167, **Calories from Fat:** 22%, **Total Fat:** 4g,
Saturated Fat: 1g, **Cholesterol:** 61mg, **Sodium:** 313mg,
Carbohydrate: 16g, **Fiber:** <1g, **Protein:** 14g

Dietary Exchange: 1 Starch, 1½ Meat

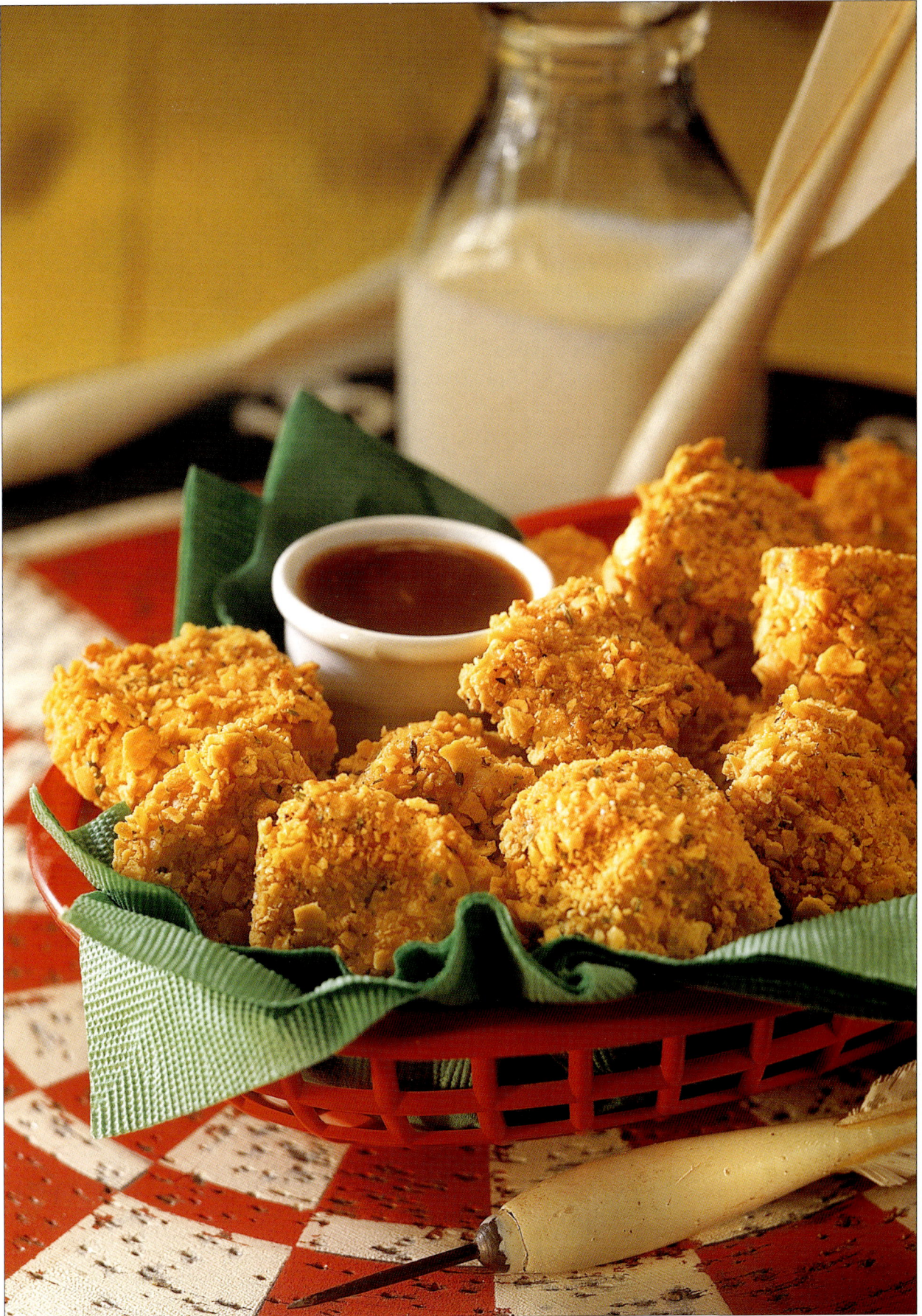

Chicken Nuggets with Barbecue Dipping Sauce

Surfin' Salmon

Makes 5 servings

- ⅓ cup cornflake crumbs
- ⅓ cup cholesterol-free egg substitute
- 2 tablespoons fat-free (skim) milk
- ¾ teaspoon dried dill weed
- ⅛ teaspoon black pepper
- Dash hot pepper sauce
- 1 (14½-ounce) can salmon, drained and skin and bones removed
- Nonstick cooking spray
- 1 teaspoon olive oil
- 6 tablespoons tartar sauce
- 5 small pieces pimiento

1. Stir together cornflake crumbs, egg substitute, milk, dill weed, black pepper and hot pepper sauce in large mixing bowl. Add salmon; mix well.

2. Shape salmon mixture into 5 large egg-shaped balls. Flatten each into ¾-inch-thick oval. Pinch one end of each oval into tail shape for fish.

3. Spray large nonstick skillet with cooking spray. Cook fish over medium-high heat 2 to 3 minutes or until lightly browned; turn. Add oil to skillet. Continue cooking 2 to 3 minutes or until firm and lightly browned.

4. Place small drop tartar sauce and pimiento on each for "eye." Serve with remaining tartar sauce, if desired.

Serving Suggestion: Serve romaine lettuce on the side of the Surfin' Salmon patty to add the look of sea plants.

Nutrients per serving: 1 Salmon patty
Calories: 279, **Calories from Fat:** 54%, **Total Fat:** 17g,
Saturated Fat: 3g, **Cholesterol:** 37mg, **Sodium:** 638mg,
Carbohydrate: 12g, **Fiber:** 2g, **Protein:** 20g

Dietary Exchange: ½ Starch, 2½ Meat, 1½ Fat

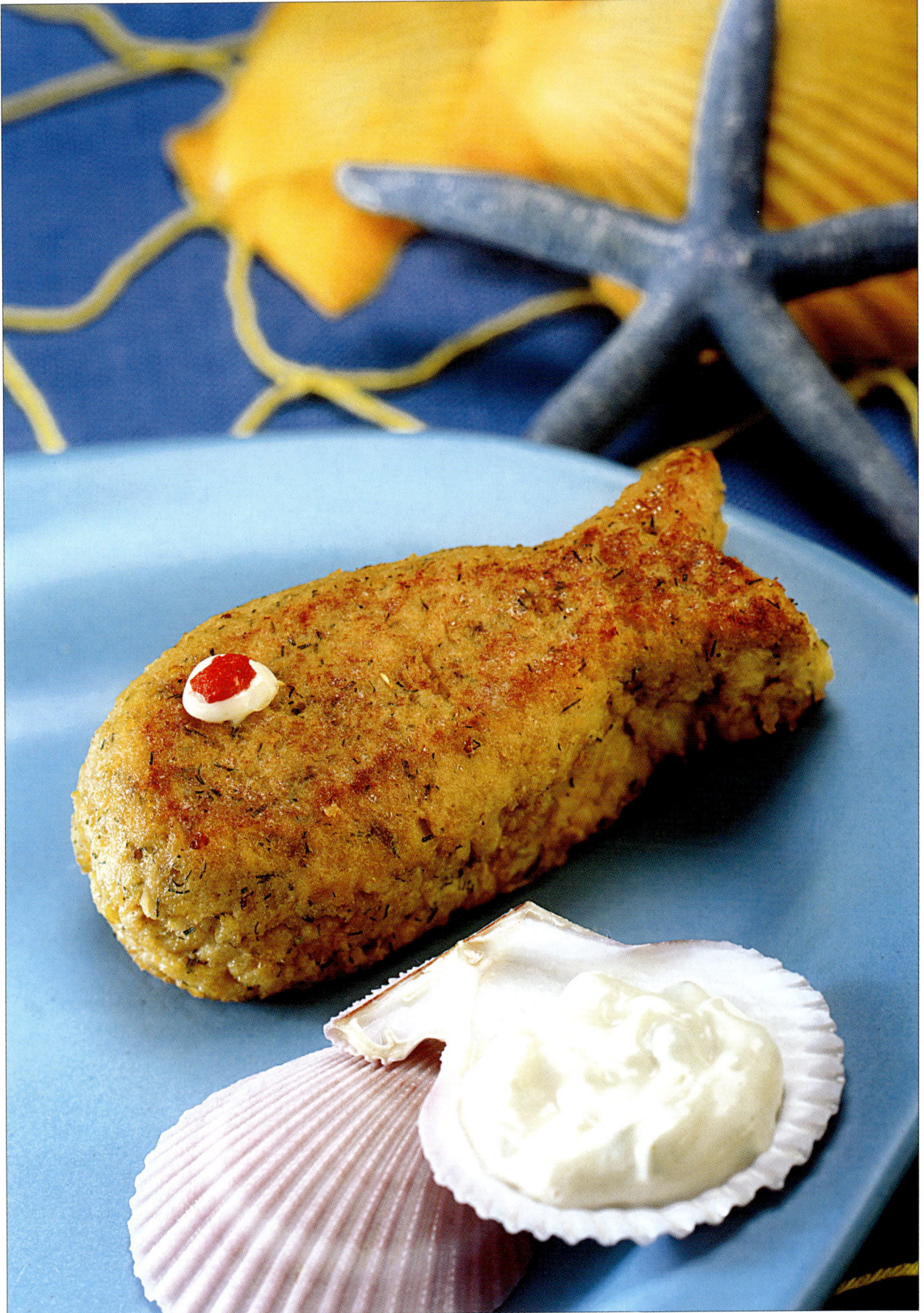

Surfin' Salmon

Double-Sauced Chicken Pizza Bagels

Makes 2 servings

>   1 (about 3½ ounces) whole bagel, split in half
>   ¼ cup prepared pizza sauce
>   ½ cup diced cooked chicken breast
>   ¼ cup (1 ounce) shredded part-skim mozzarella cheese
>   2 teaspoons grated Parmesan cheese

1. Place bagel halves on microwavable plate.

2. Spoon 1 tablespoon pizza sauce onto each bagel half. Spread evenly using back of spoon.

3. Top each bagel half with ¼ cup chicken. Spoon 1 tablespoon pizza sauce over chicken on each bagel half.

4. Sprinkle 2 tablespoons mozzarella cheese over top of each bagel half.

5. Cover bagel halves loosely with waxed paper; microwave at HIGH 1 to 1½ minutes or until cheese melts.

6. Carefully remove waxed paper. Sprinkle each bagel half with 1 teaspoon Parmesan cheese. Let stand 1 minute before serving to cool slightly. (Bagels will be very hot.)

Tip: For crunchier "pizzas," toast bagels before adding toppings.

Nutrients per serving: 1 Bagel half
Calories: 231, **Calories from Fat:** 23%, **Total Fat:** 5g,
Saturated Fat: 3g, **Cholesterol:** 32mg, **Sodium:** 390mg,
Carbohydrate: 31g, **Fiber:** 2g, **Protein:** 18g

Dietary Exchange: 2 Starch, 1½ Meat

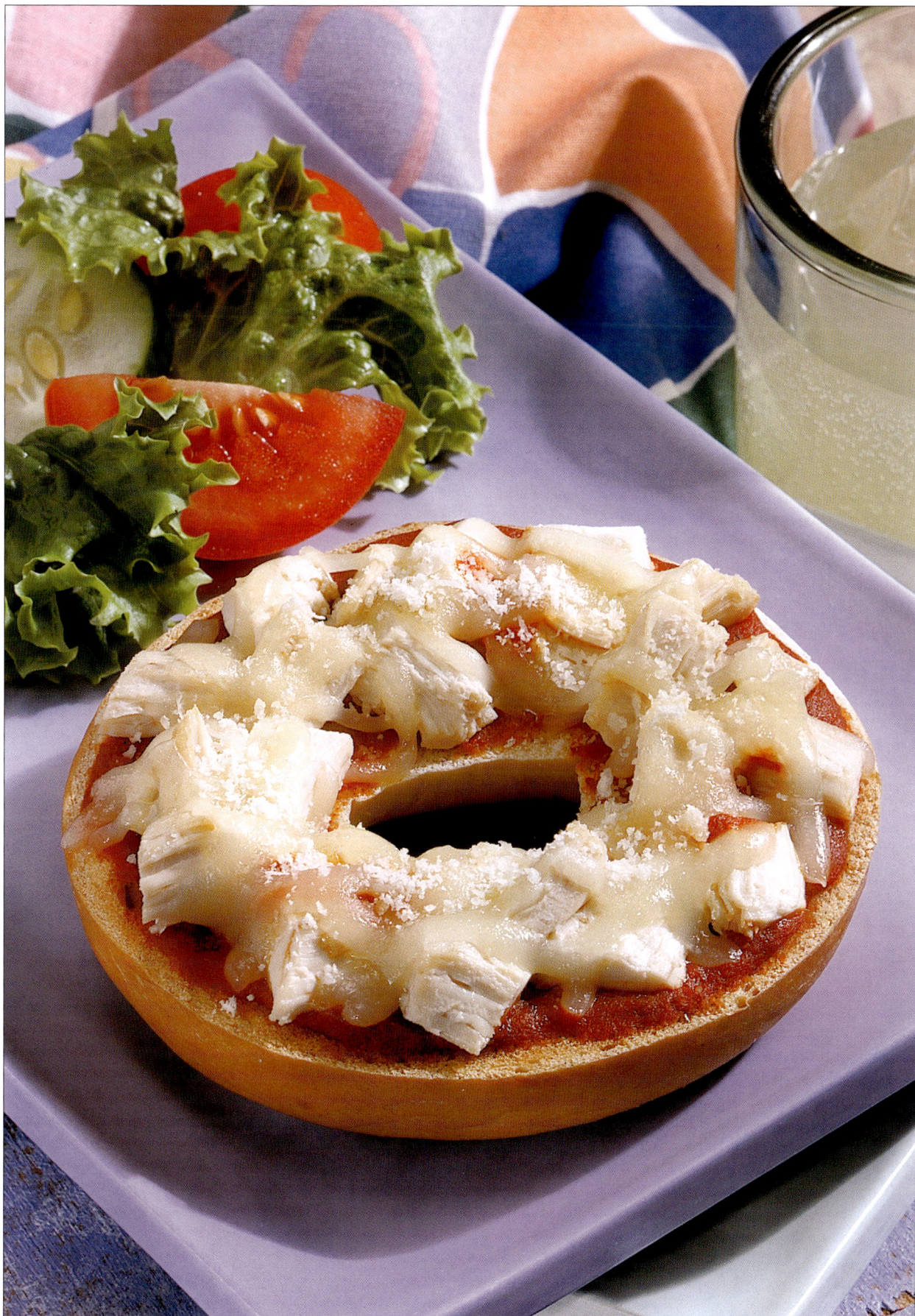

Double-Sauced Chicken Pizza Bagel

Peanut Butter-Pineapple Celery Sticks

Makes 6 servings

- ½ **cup low-fat (1%) cottage cheese**
- ½ **cup reduced-fat peanut butter**
- ½ **cup crushed pineapple in juice, drained**
- 12 **(3-inch-long) celery sticks**

Combine cottage cheese and peanut butter in food processor. Blend until smooth. Stir in pineapple. Stuff celery sticks with mixture.

Serving Suggestion: Substitute 2 medium apples, sliced, for celery.

Travel Tip: Place ¼ cup Peanut Butter-Pineapple filling in small plastic container. Cover. Pack container and celery sticks wrapped in plastic wrap in bag with small ice pack.

Nutrients per serving: 2 Celery Sticks with ¼ cup Peanut Butter-Pineapple filling
Calories: 165, **Calories from Fat:** 43%, **Total Fat:** 8g, **Saturated Fat:** 2g, **Cholesterol:** 1mg, **Sodium:** 313mg, **Carbohydrate:** 17g, **Fiber:** 3g, **Protein:** 8g

Dietary Exchange: 1 Fruit, 1 Meat, 1 Fat

Tuna Melt

Makes 4 servings

> 1 **can (12 ounces) chunk white tuna packed in water, drained and flaked**
> 1½ **cups coleslaw mix**
> 3 **tablespoons sliced green onions**
> 3 **tablespoons reduced-fat mayonnaise**
> 1 **tablespoon Dijon mustard**
> 1 **teaspoon dried dill weed**
> 4 **English muffins, split and lightly toasted**
> ⅓ **cup shredded reduced-fat Cheddar cheese**

1. Preheat broiler. Combine tuna, coleslaw mix and green onions in medium bowl. Combine mayonnaise, mustard and dill weed in small bowl. Stir mayonnaise mixture into tuna mixture. Spread tuna mixture onto muffin halves. Place on broiler pan.

2. Broil 4 inches from heat 3 to 4 minutes or until heated through. Sprinkle with cheese. Broil 1 to 2 minutes more or until cheese melts.

Nutrients per serving: 2 Melts
Calories: 313, **Calories from Fat:** 23%, **Total Fat:** 8g,
Saturated Fat: 2g, **Cholesterol:** 43mg, **Sodium:** 882mg,
Carbohydrate: 30g, **Fiber:** 2g, **Protein:** 30g

Dietary Exchange: 2 Starch, 3 Meat

snacking sensations

Wild Wedges

Makes 4 servings

> 2 (8-inch) fat-free flour tortillas
>   Nonstick cooking spray
> ⅓ cup shredded reduced-fat Cheddar cheese
> ⅓ cup chopped cooked chicken or turkey
> 1 green onion, thinly sliced
> 2 tablespoons mild, thick and chunky salsa

1. Heat large nonstick skillet over medium heat until hot.

2. Spray one side of one flour tortilla with cooking spray; place, sprayed side down, in skillet. Top with cheese, chicken, green onion and salsa. Place remaining tortilla over mixture; spray with cooking spray.

3. Cook 2 to 3 minutes per side or until golden brown and cheese is melted. Cut into 8 triangles.

Variation: For bean quesadillas, omit the chicken and spread ⅓ cup canned fat-free refried beans over one of the tortillas.

Nutrients per serving: 2 Wedges (made with chicken)
Calories: 76, **Calories from Fat:** 24%, **Total Fat:** 2g,
Saturated Fat: 1g, **Cholesterol:** 14mg, **Sodium:** 282mg,
Carbohydrate: 8g, **Fiber:** 4g, **Protein:** 7g

Dietary Exchange: ½ Starch, 1 Meat

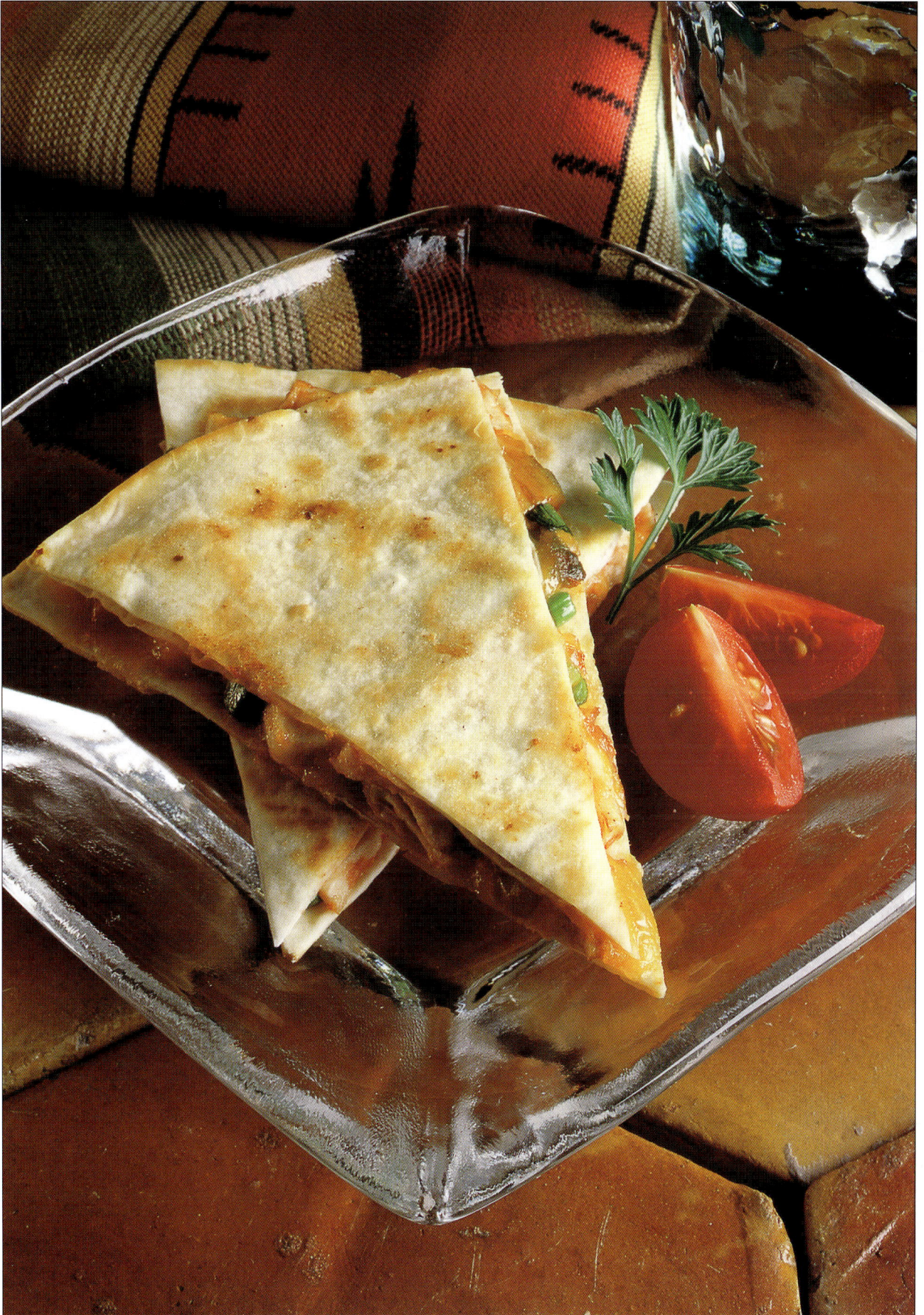

Wild Wedges

Tooty Fruitys

Makes 10 servings

- 1 **package (10 ounces) extra-light flaky biscuits**
- 10 **(1½-inch) fruit pieces, such as plum, apple, peach or pear pieces**
- 1 **egg white**
- 1 **teaspoon water**
  Powdered sugar (optional)

1. Preheat oven to 425°F. Spray baking sheets with nonstick cooking spray; set aside.

2. Separate biscuits. Place on lightly floured surface. Roll with lightly floured rolling pin or flatten dough with fingers to form 3½-inch circles. Place 1 fruit piece in center of each circle. Bring 3 edges of dough up over fruit; pinch edges together to seal. Place on prepared baking sheet.

3. Beat egg white with water in small bowl; brush over dough.

4. Bake until golden brown, 10 to 15 minutes. Remove to wire rack to cool. Serve warm or at room temperature. Sprinkle with powdered sugar, if desired, just before serving.

Cheesy Tooty Fruitys: Prepare dough circles as directed. Top each circle with ½ teaspoon softened reduced-fat cream cheese in addition to the fruit. Continue as directed.

Nutrients per serving: 1 Tooty Fruity
Calories: 93, **Calories from Fat:** 24%, **Total Fat:** 3g,
Saturated Fat: <1g, **Cholesterol:** 0mg, **Sodium:** 230mg,
Carbohydrate: 16g, **Fiber:** 1g, **Protein:** 2g

Dietary Exchange: ½ Starch, ½ Fruit, ½ Fat

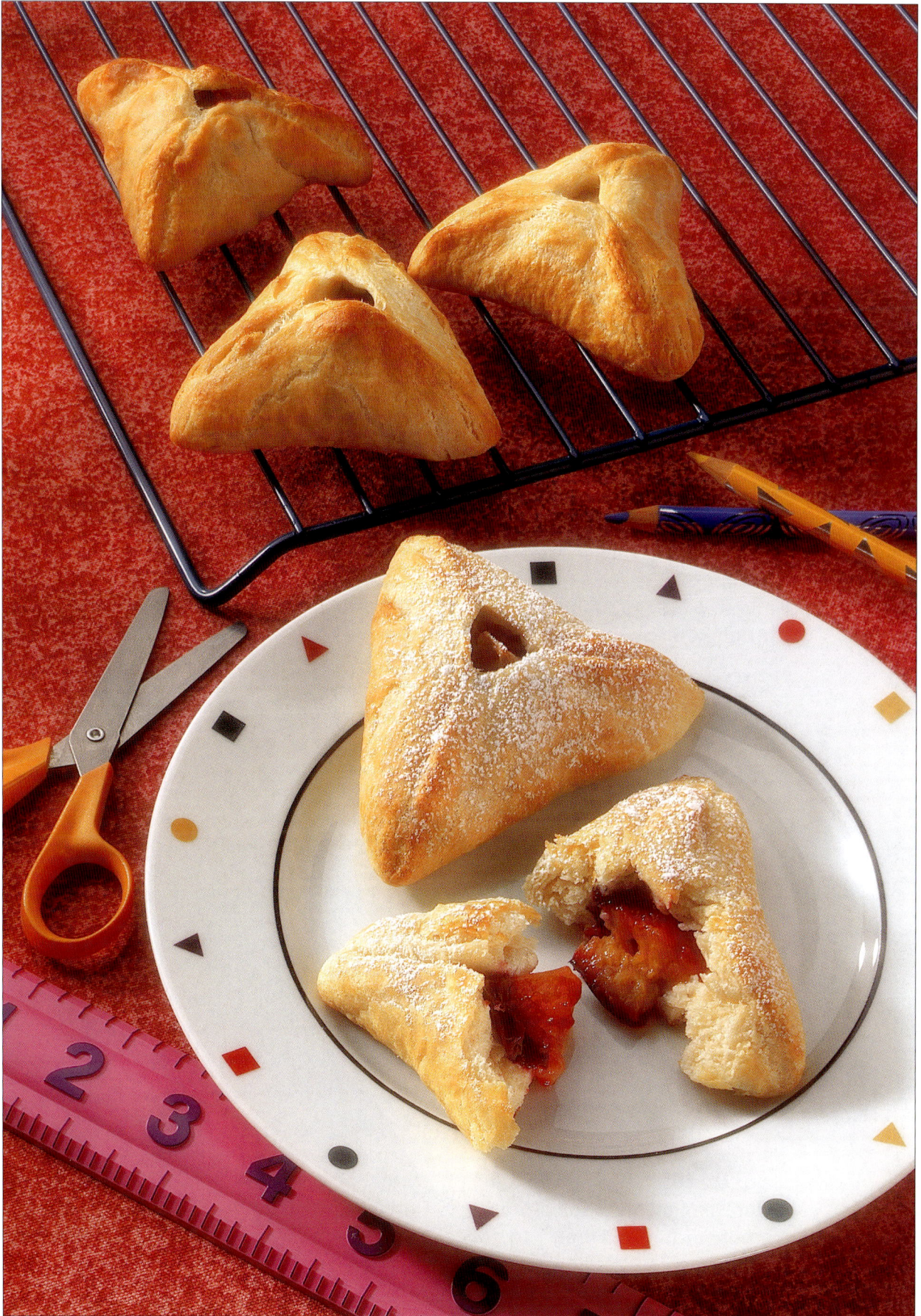

Tooty Fruitys

67

Cheesy Barbecued Bean Dip

Makes 4 servings

- ½ cup canned vegetarian baked beans
- 3 tablespoons pasteurized process cheese spread
- 2 tablespoons regular or hickory smoke barbecue sauce
  Green onions (optional)
- 2 large carrots, cut into diagonal slices
- 1 medium red or green bell pepper, cut into chunks

1. Place beans in small microwavable bowl; mash with fork. Stir in cheese spread and barbecue sauce. Cover with vented plastic wrap.

2. Microwave at HIGH 1 minute; stir. Microwave 30 seconds or until hot. Garnish with green onion and bell pepper cutouts, if desired. Serve with carrot slices and bell pepper chunks.

Nutrients per serving:
Calories: 93, **Calories from Fat:** 25%, **Total Fat:** 3g,
Saturated Fat: 1g, **Cholesterol:** 10mg, **Sodium:** 355mg,
Carbohydrate: 15g, **Fiber:** 4g, **Protein:** 4g

Dietary Exchange: 1 Starch, ½ Fat

Cheesy Chips

Makes 4 servings

- 10 wonton wrappers
- 2 tablespoons powdered American cheese or grated
    Parmesan cheese
- 2 teaspoons olive oil
- ⅛ teaspoon garlic powder

1. Preheat oven to 375°F. Spray baking sheet with nonstick cooking spray. Diagonally cut each wonton wrapper in half, forming two triangles. Place in single layer on prepared baking sheet.

2. Combine cheese, oil and garlic powder in small bowl. Sprinkle over wonton triangles. Bake 6 to 8 minutes or until golden brown and crisp. Remove from oven. Cool completely.

Nutrients per serving: 5 Chips
Calories: 75, **Calories from Fat:** 38%, **Total Fat:** 3g,
Saturated Fat: 1g, **Cholesterol:** 4mg, **Sodium:** 92mg,
Carbohydrate: 9g, **Fiber:** <1g, **Protein:** 2g

Dietary Exchange: ½ Starch, ½ Fat

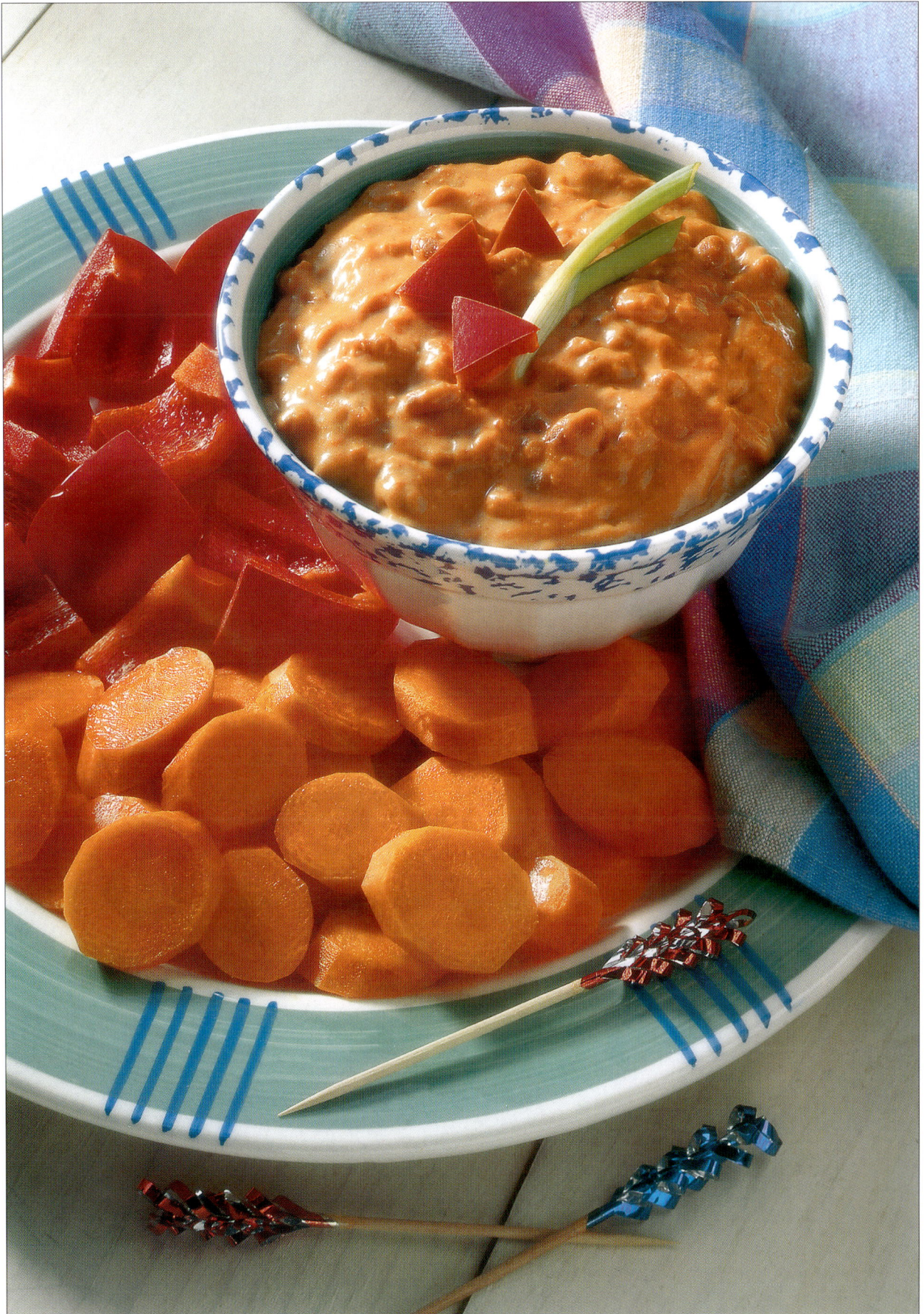
Cheesy Barbecued Bean Dip

snackingsensations

Confetti Tuna in Celery Sticks

Makes 10 to 12 servings

- 1 (3-ounce) pouch of STARKIST® Premium Albacore or Chunk Light Tuna
- ½ cup shredded red or green cabbage
- ½ cup shredded carrot
- ¼ cup shredded yellow squash or zucchini
- 3 tablespoons reduced-calorie cream cheese, softened
- 1 tablespoon plain low-fat yogurt
- ½ teaspoon dried basil, crushed
  Salt and pepper to taste
- 10 to 12 (4-inch) celery sticks, with leaves if desired

1. In a small bowl toss together tuna, cabbage, carrot and squash. Stir in cream cheese, yogurt and basil. Add salt and pepper to taste.

2. With small spatula spread mixture evenly into celery sticks.

Prep Time: 20 minutes

Nutrients per serving: 1 (4-inch) Celery Stick filled with about 3 tablespoons Tuna mixture
Calories: 32, **Calories from Fat:** 26%, **Total Fat:** 1g, **Saturated Fat:** 1g, **Cholesterol:** 5mg, **Sodium:** 90mg, **Carbohydrate:** 3g, **Fiber:** 1g, **Protein:** 3g

Dietary Exchange: ½ Meat

Peanutty Banana Dip

Makes ¾ cup

- ½ cup sliced bananas
- ⅓ cup reduced-fat creamy peanut butter
- 2 tablespoons fat-free (skim) milk
- 1 tablespoon honey
- ½ teaspoon vanilla
- ⅛ teaspoon ground cinnamon

Place all ingredients in blender and process until smooth.

Tip: Try the dip with Granny Smith apple slices or celery sticks.

Nutrients per serving: 1 tablespoon Dip
Calories: 54, **Calories from Fat:** 42%, **Total Fat:** 3g, **Saturated Fat:** <1g, **Cholesterol:** <1mg, **Sodium:** 57mg, **Carbohydrate:** 5g, **Fiber:** <1g, **Protein:** 2g

Dietary Exchange: ½ Fruit, ½ Fat

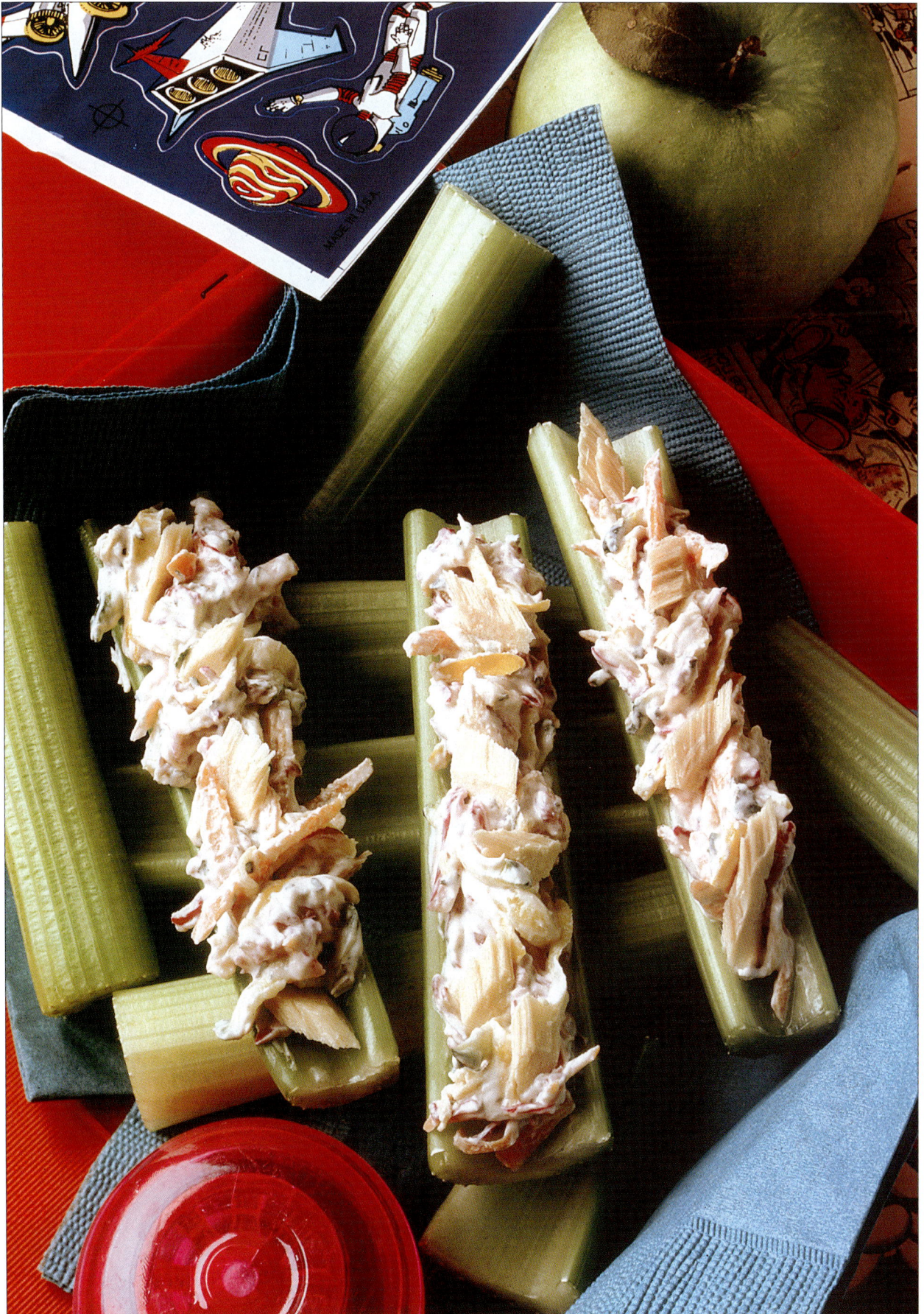

Confetti Tuna in Celery Sticks

Easy Nachos

Makes 4 servings

- 4 **(6-inch) flour tortillas**
  Nonstick cooking spray
- 4 **ounces lean ground turkey**
- ⅔ **cup salsa (mild or medium)**
- 2 **tablespoons sliced green onion**
- ½ **cup (2 ounces) shredded reduced-fat Cheddar cheese**

1. Preheat oven to 350°F. Cut each tortilla into 8 wedges; lightly spray one side of wedges with cooking spray. Place on ungreased baking sheet. Bake 5 to 9 minutes or until lightly browned and crisp.

2. Meanwhile, cook ground turkey in small nonstick skillet until browned, stirring with spoon to break up meat. Drain fat. Stir in salsa. Cook until hot.

3. Sprinkle meat mixture over tortilla wedges. Sprinkle with green onion. Top with cheese. Return to oven 1 to 2 minutes or until cheese melts.

Serving Suggestion: Cut tortillas into shapes with cookie cutters and bake as directed.

Tip: In a hurry? Substitute baked corn chips for flour tortillas and cooking spray. Proceed as directed.

Nutrients per serving: 8 Nachos
Calories: 209, **Calories from Fat:** 32%, **Total Fat:** 7g,
Saturated Fat: 2g, **Cholesterol:** 29mg, **Sodium:** 703mg,
Carbohydrate: 23g, **Fiber:** 2g, **Protein:** 12g

Dietary Exchange: 1 Starch, 1 Vegetable, 1 Meat, 1 Fat

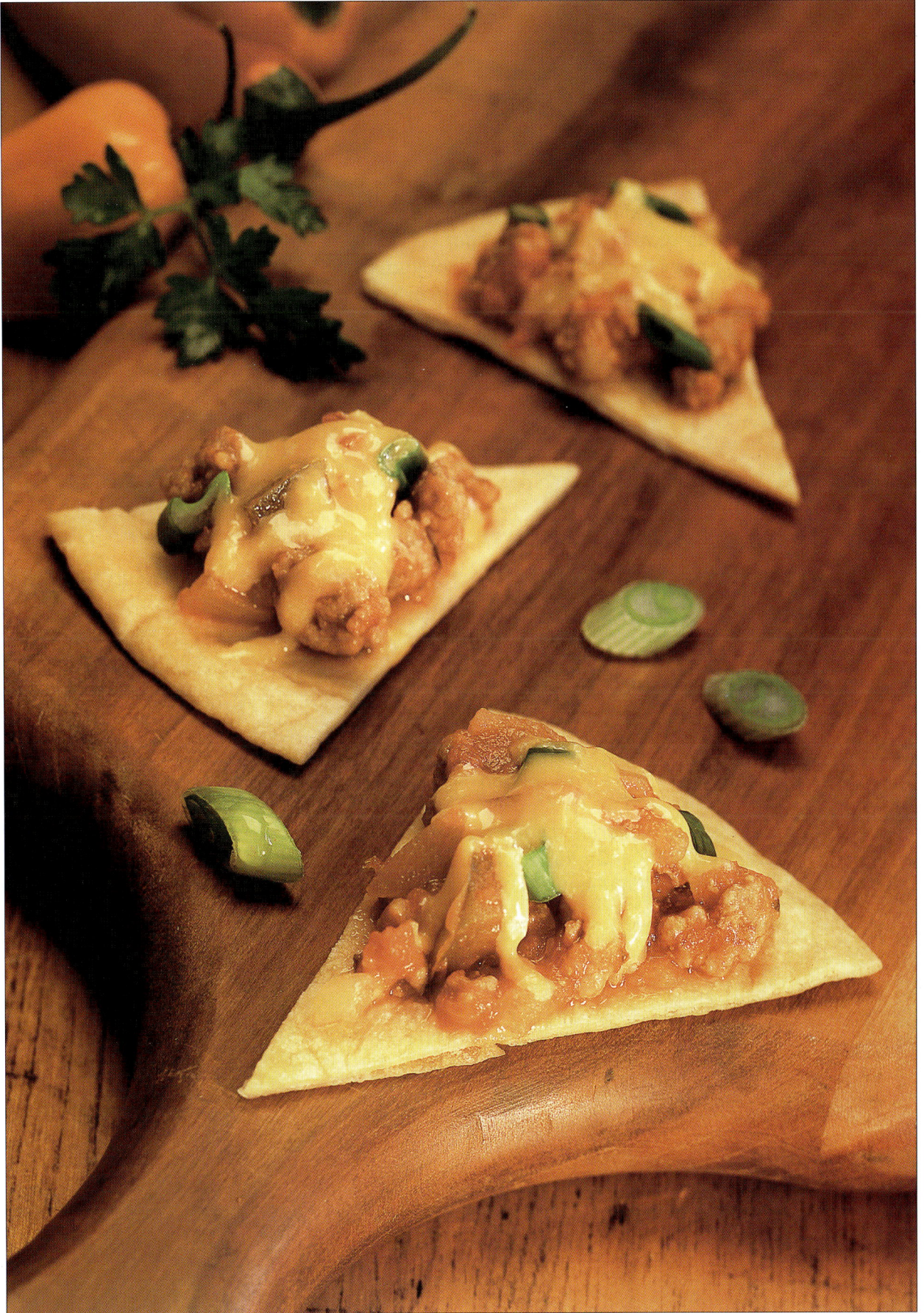

Easy Nachos

Curly Lettuce Wrappers

Makes 4 servings

- 4 green leaf lettuce leaves
- ¼ cup reduced-fat sour cream
- 4 turkey bacon slices, crisp-cooked and crumbled
- ½ cup (2 ounces) crumbled feta or blue cheese
- 8 ounces thinly sliced deli turkey breast
- 4 whole green onions
- ½ medium red or green bell pepper, thinly sliced
- 1 cup broccoli sprouts

1. Rinse lettuce leaves and pat dry.

2. Combine sour cream and bacon in small bowl. Spread ¼ of sour cream mixture evenly over center third of one lettuce leaf. Sprinkle 2 tablespoons cheese over sour cream. Top with 2 ounces turkey.

3. Cut off green portion of each green onion, reserving white onion bottoms for another use. Place green portion of 1 onion, ¼ of bell pepper slices and ¼ cup sprouts on top of turkey.

4. Fold right edge of lettuce over filling; fold bottom edge up over filling. Loosely roll up from folded right edge, leaving left edge of wrap open. Repeat with remaining ingredients.

Travel Tip: Wrap individually in plastic wrap. Store in cooler with ice.

Nutrients per serving: 1 Lettuce Wrapper
Calories: 155, **Calories from Fat:** 41%, **Total Fat:** 7g,
Saturated Fat: 4g, **Cholesterol:** 75mg, **Sodium:** 987mg,
Carbohydrate: 6g, **Fiber:** <1g, **Protein:** 17g

Dietary Exchange: 1 Vegetable, 2 Meat, ½ Fat

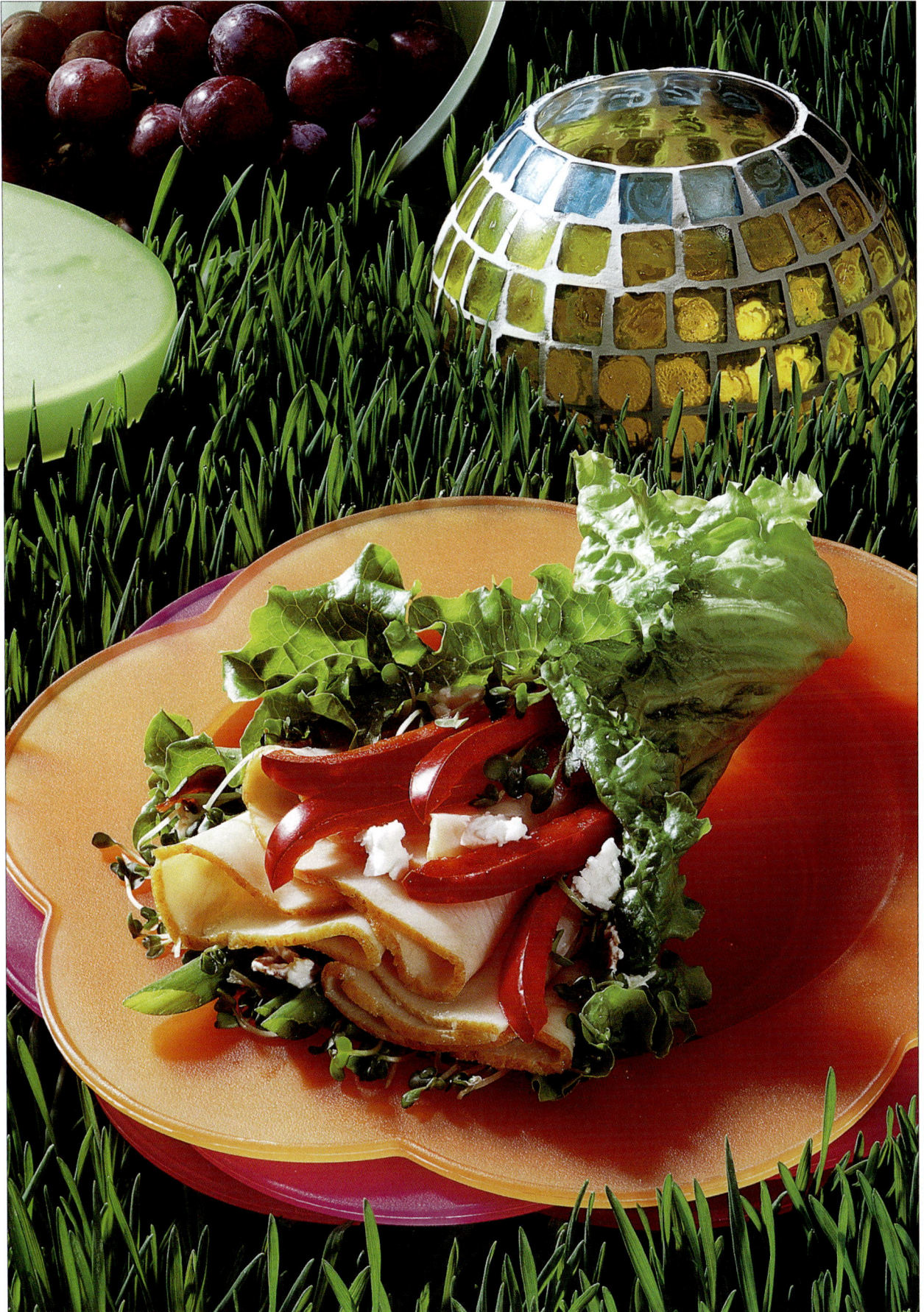

Curly Lettuce Wrapper

delicious
desserts

Chocolate Rum Bread Pudding

Makes 9 servings

- 2 **eggs**
- 1 **egg white**
- 2½ **cups fat-free milk**
- ¼ **cup spiced rum**
- 3 **tablespoons unsweetened cocoa powder**
- 15 **packets NatraTaste® Brand Sugar Substitute**
- 1 **teaspoon vanilla**
- 4 **cups dry Italian or French bread cubes**

1. Preheat oven to 350°F. Coat a 9-inch deep-dish baking pan with nonstick cooking spray.

2. Combine first 7 ingredients (eggs through vanilla) in a blender, and process until smooth. Spread the bread cubes in the pan. Pour the milk mixture over the bread cubes. Press down on the bread with a spoon. Set aside for 10 minutes. Bake 40 minutes, or until knife inserted in center comes out clean. Serve with Papaya Guava Dessert Sauce (recipe follows).

Papaya Guava Dessert Sauce: Combine 1½ cups cubed papaya, ¾ cup frozen guava pulp, thawed, 9 ounces unsweetened pineapple juice and 6 packets NutraTaste® Brand Sugar Substitute in a blender; process until smooth. Serve at room temperature.

Nutrients per serving:
Calories: 140, **Calories from Fat:** 13%, **Total Fat:** 2g, **Saturated Fat:** <1g, **Cholesterol:** 50mg, **Sodium:** 145mg, **Carbohydrate:** 21g, **Fiber:** 3g, **Protein:** 7g

Dietary Exchange: 1 Starch, ½ Fruit, ½ Fat

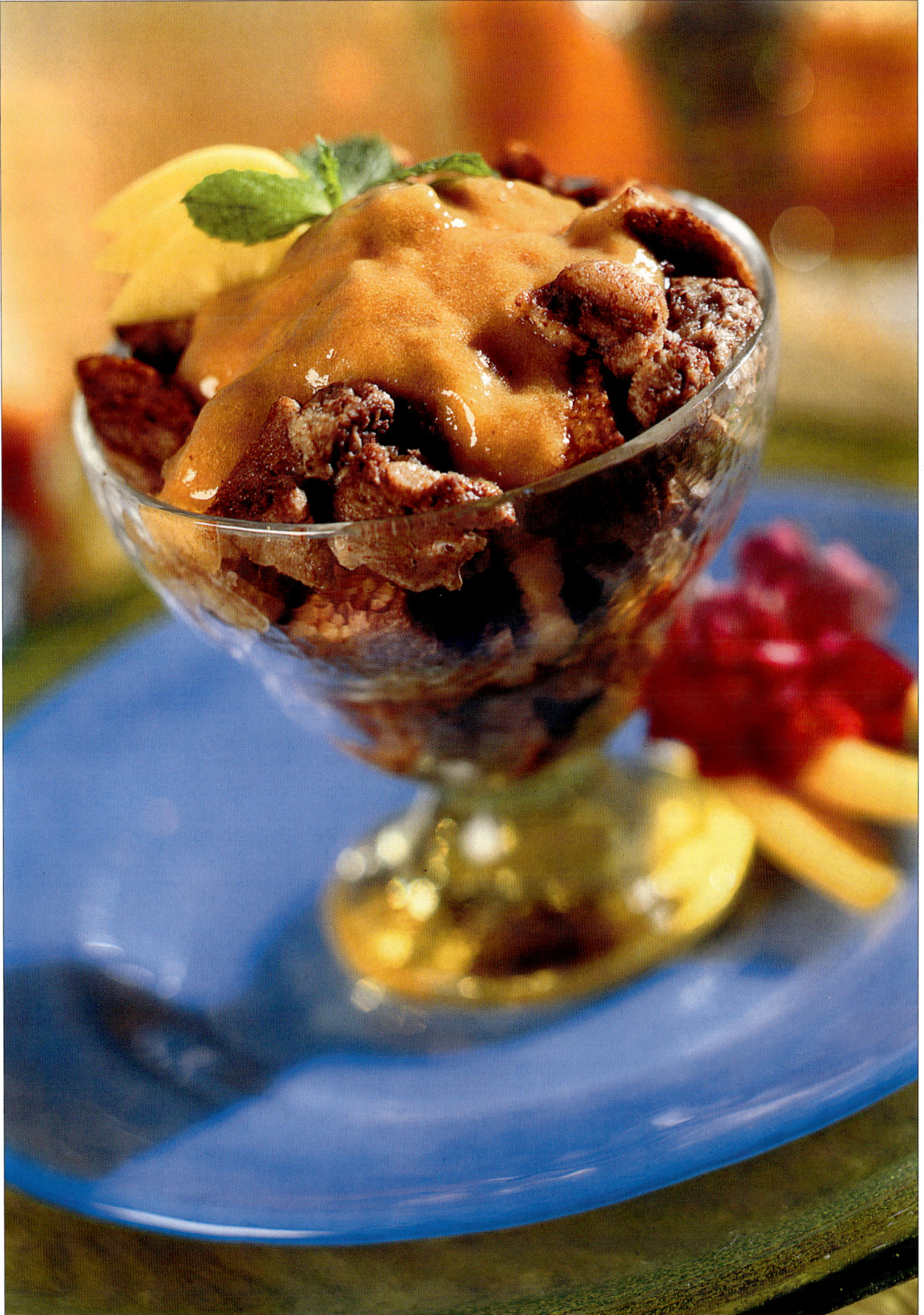

Chocolate Rum Bread Pudding

Hidden Pumpkin Pies

Makes 6 servings

- 1½ **cups canned solid-pack pumpkin**
- 1 **cup evaporated skimmed milk**
- ½ **cup cholesterol-free egg substitute**
- ¼ **cup no-calorie sweetener**
- 1 **teaspoon pumpkin pie spice***
- 1¼ **teaspoons vanilla, divided**
- 3 **egg whites**
- ¼ **teaspoon cream of tartar**
- ⅓ **cup honey**

Substitute ½ teaspoon ground cinnamon, ¼ teaspoon ground ginger and ⅛ teaspoon each ground allspice and ground nutmeg for 1 teaspoon pumpkin pie spice.

1. Preheat oven to 350°F.

2. Stir together pumpkin, evaporated milk, egg substitute, sweetener, pumpkin pie spice and 1 teaspoon vanilla. Pour into 6 (6-ounce) custard cups or 6 (¾-cup) soufflé dishes. Place in shallow baking dish or pan. Pour boiling water around custard cups to depth of 1 inch. Bake 25 minutes.

3. Meanwhile, beat egg whites, cream of tartar and remaining ¼ teaspoon vanilla at high speed of electric mixer until soft peaks form. Gradually add honey, beating until stiff peaks form.

4. Spread egg white mixture on top of hot pumpkin mixture. Return to oven. Bake 15 to 16 minutes or until tops are golden brown. Let stand 10 minutes. Serve warm.

Nutrients per serving: 1 Pie
Calories: 148, **Calories from Fat:** 10%, **Total Fat:** 2g,
Saturated Fat: 1g, **Cholesterol:** 54mg, **Sodium:** 133mg,
Carbohydrate: 27g, **Fiber:** 2g, **Protein:** 8g

Dietary Exchange: 1½ Starch, 1 Meat

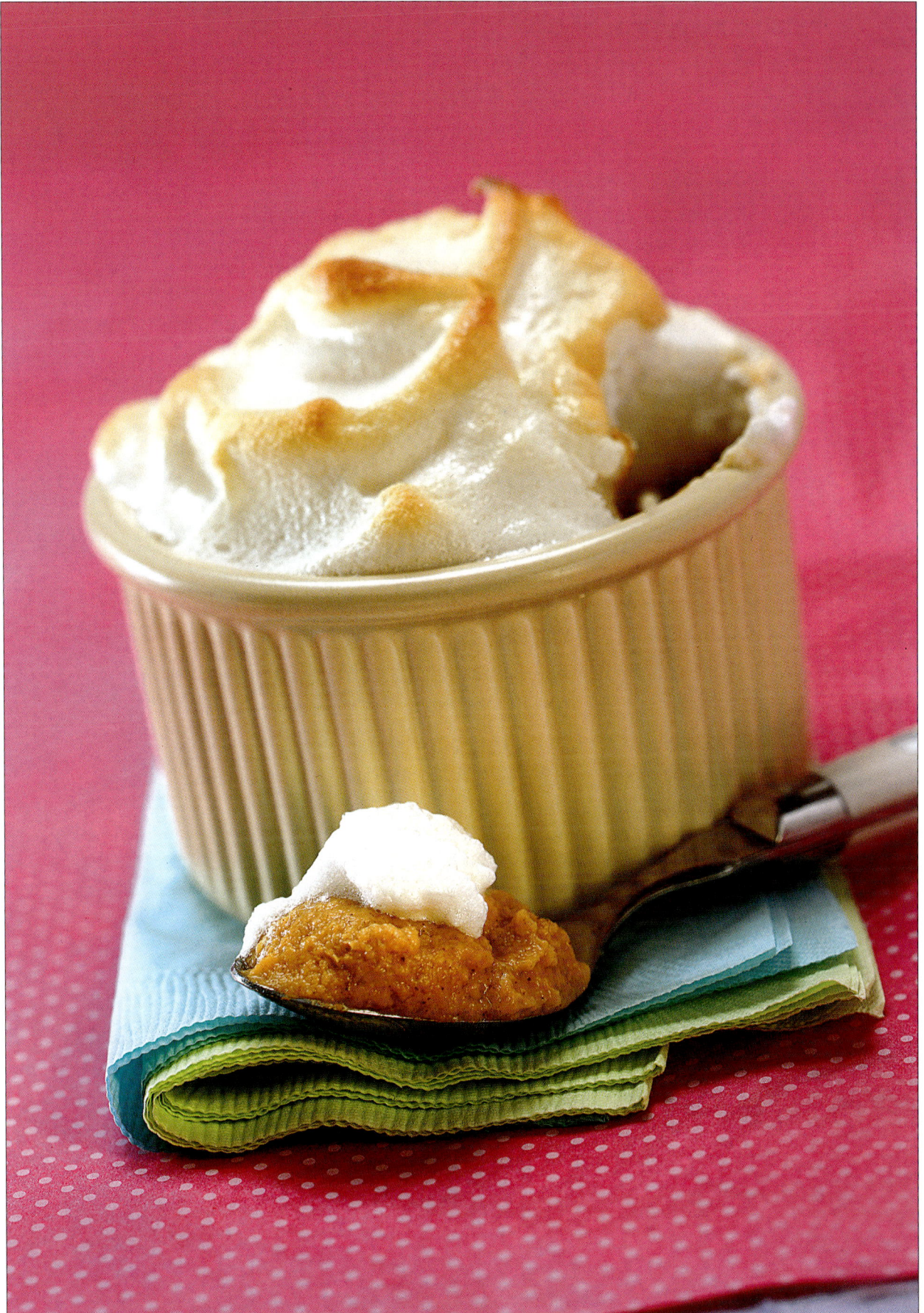

Hidden Pumpkin Pie

Cream Cheese Brownie Royale

Makes 16 servings

- 1 package (about 15 ounces) low-fat brownie mix
- ⅔ cup cold coffee or water
- 1 package (8 ounces) reduced-fat cream cheese, softened
- ¼ cup fat-free (skim) milk
- 5 packets sugar substitute *or* equivalent of 10 teaspoons sugar
- ½ teaspoon vanilla

1. Preheat oven to 350°F. Coat 13×9-inch nonstick baking pan with nonstick cooking spray.

2. Combine brownie mix and coffee in large bowl; stir until blended. Pour brownie mixture into prepared pan.

3. Beat cream cheese, milk, sugar substitute and vanilla in medium bowl with electric mixer at medium speed until smooth. Spoon cream cheese mixture in dollops over brownie mixture. Swirl cream cheese mixture into brownie mixture with tip of knife.

4. Bake 30 to 35 minutes or until toothpick inserted in center comes out clean. Cool completely in pan on wire rack.

5. Cover with foil and refrigerate 8 hours or until ready to serve. Cut into 16 squares; garnish as desired.

Nutrients per serving: 1 Brownie
Calories: 167, **Calories from Fat:** 25%, **Total Fat:** 5g,
Saturated Fat: 2g, **Cholesterol:** 7mg, **Sodium:** 181mg,
Carbohydrate: 28g, **Fiber:** 1g, **Protein:** 4g

Dietary Exchange: 2 Starch, ½ Fat

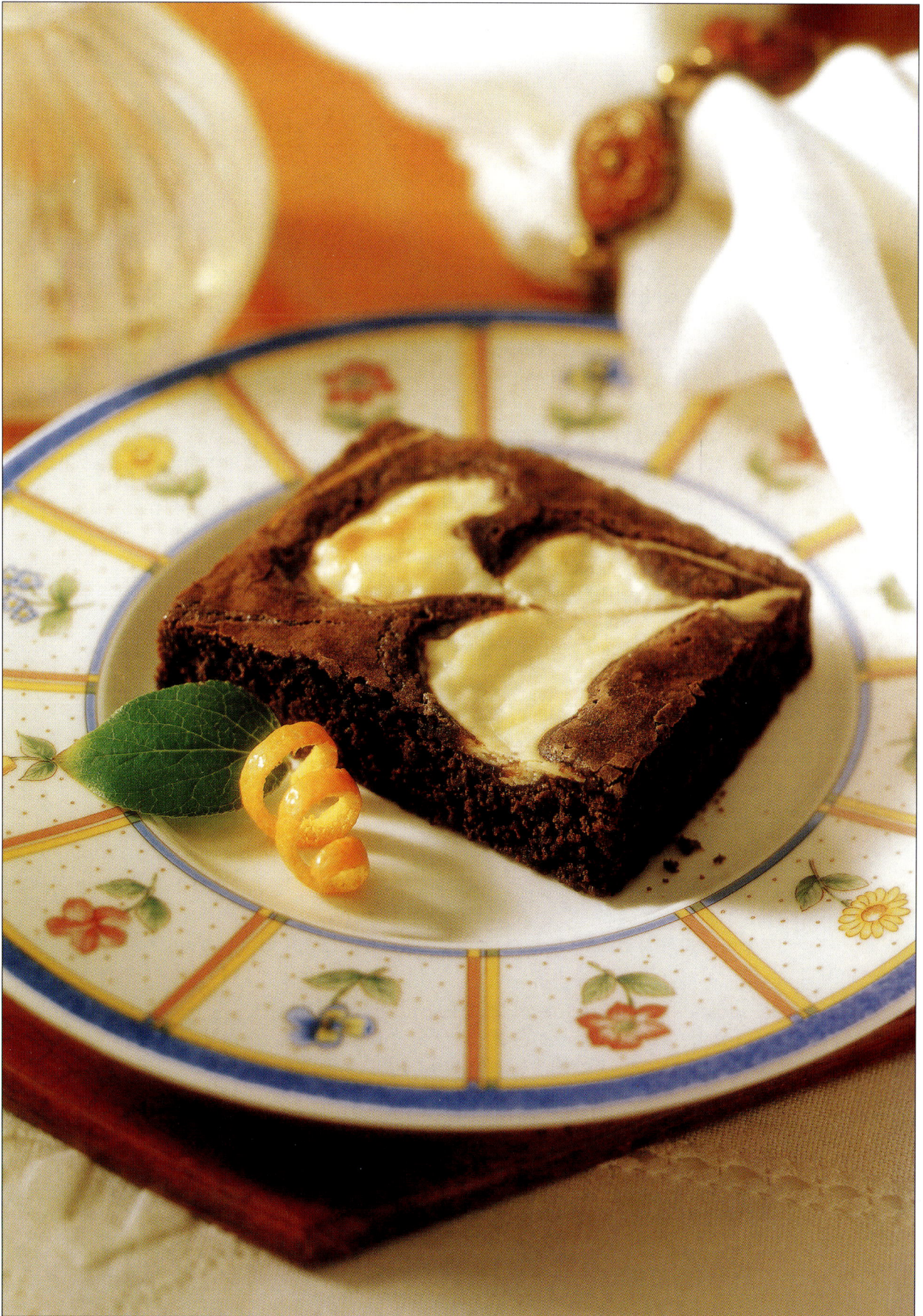

Cream Cheese Brownie Royale

Chocolate-Almond Meringue Puffs

Makes 15 servings

2	tablespoons granulated sugar
3	packets sugar substitute
1½	teaspoons unsweetened cocoa powder
2	egg whites, at room temperature
½	teaspoon vanilla
¼	teaspoon cream of tartar
¼	teaspoon almond extract
⅛	teaspoon salt
1½	ounces sliced almonds
3	tablespoons sugar-free seedless raspberry fruit spread

1. Preheat oven to 275°F. Combine granulated sugar, sugar substitute and cocoa powder in small bowl; set aside.

2. Place egg whites in small bowl; beat at high speed of electric mixer until foamy. Add vanilla, cream of tartar, almond extract and salt; beat until soft peaks form. Add sugar mixture, 1 tablespoon at a time, beating until stiff peaks form.

3. Line baking sheet with foil. Spoon 15 equal mounds of egg white mixture onto foil. Sprinkle with almonds.

4. Bake 1 hour. Turn oven off but do not open door. Leave puffs in oven 2 hours longer or until completely dry. Remove from oven; cool completely.

5. Stir fruit spread and spoon about ½ teaspoon onto each meringue just before serving.

Tip: Puffs are best if eaten the same day they're made. If necessary, store in airtight container, adding fruit topping at time of serving.

Nutrients per serving: 1 Puff
Calories: 34, **Calories from Fat:** 26%, **Total Fat:** 1g,
Saturated Fat: 0g, **Cholesterol:** 0mg, **Sodium:** 27mg,
Carbohydrate: 4g, **Fiber:** <1g, **Protein:** 1g

Dietary Exchange: ½ Starch

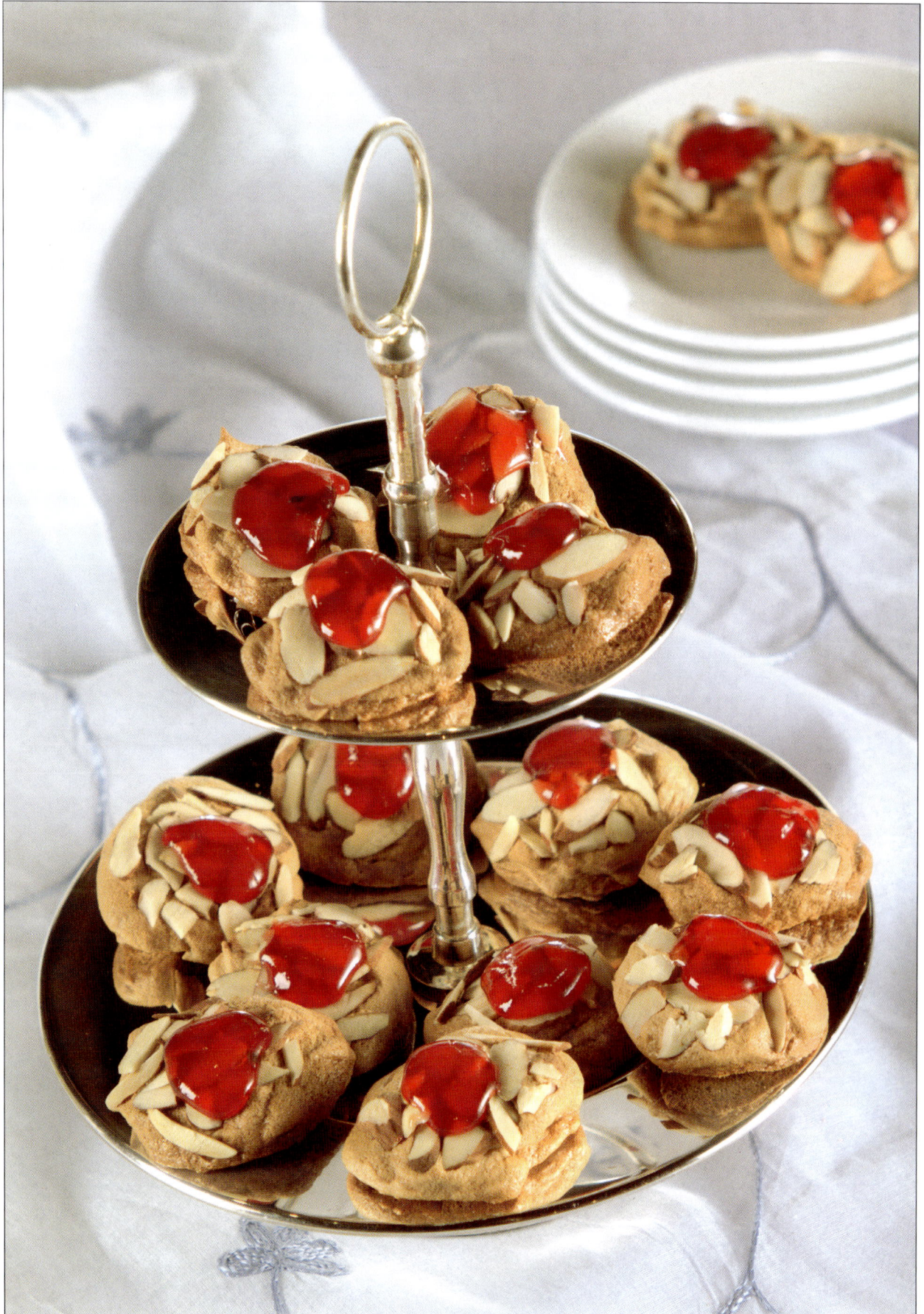

Chocolate-Almond Meringue Puffs

deliciousdesserts

Caffé en Forchetta

Makes 6 servings

> 2 **cups reduced-fat (2%) milk**
> 1 **cup cholesterol-free egg substitute**
> ½ **cup sugar**
> 2 **tablespoons no-sugar-added mocha-flavored instant coffee**
> **Grated chocolate *or* 6 chocolate-covered coffee beans (optional)**

1. Preheat oven to 325°F.

2. Combine all ingredients except grated chocolate in medium bowl. Whisk until instant coffee has dissolved and mixture is foamy. Pour into 6 individual custard cups. Place cups in 13×9-inch baking pan. Fill pan with hot water halfway up sides of cups.

3. Bake 55 to 60 minutes or until knife inserted halfway between center and edge comes out clean. Serve warm or at room temperature. Garnish with grated chocolate or chocolate-covered coffee beans, if desired.

Note: Enjoy your dinner coffee a whole new way. Translated from Italian, Caffé en Forchetta literally means "coffee on a fork." However, a spoon is recommended when serving this wonderfully creamy dessert.

Nutrients per serving: 1 custard cupful Caffé en Forchetta (⅙ of total recipe) without garnish
Calories: 111, **Calories from Fat:** 16%, **Total Fat:** 2g,
Saturated Fat: 1g, **Cholesterol:** 6mg, **Sodium:** 136mg,
Carbohydrate: 17g, **Fiber:** 0g, **Protein:** 7g

Dietary Exchange: 1 Starch, 1 Meat

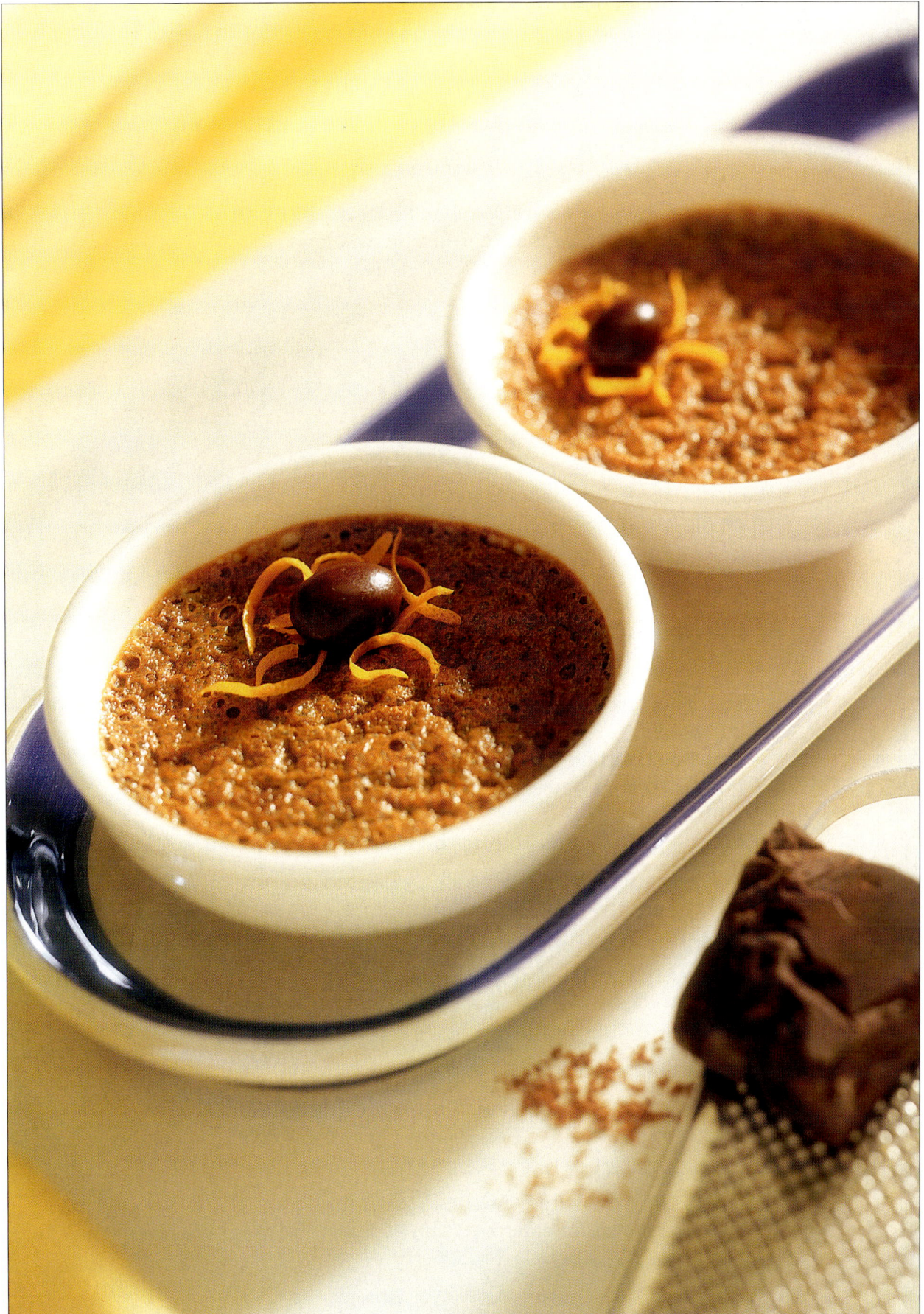

Caffé en Forchetta

deliciousdesserts

Blackberry Sorbet

Makes 2 (¾-cup) servings

> 1 (8-fluid-ounce) can chilled Vanilla GLUCERNA® Shake
> 1 cup frozen whole blackberries, unsweetened
> ½ teaspoon cinnamon
> ¼ teaspoon nutmeg
>   Sugar substitute to taste

1. In blender, combine all ingredients. Blend until thick.

2. Serve immediately or freeze 10 to 15 minutes.

Nutrients per serving: ¾ cup Sorbet
Calories: 161, **Calories from Fat:** 31%, **Total Fat:** 6g,
Saturated Fat: 1g, **Cholesterol:** 1mg, **Sodium:** 106mg,
Carbohydrate: 23g, **Fiber:** 5g, **Protein:** 6g

Dietary Exchange: 1 Starch, 1 Fruit, 1 Fat

Iced Cappuccino

Makes 2 servings

> 1 cup fat-free vanilla frozen yogurt or fat-free vanilla ice cream
> 1 cup cold strong-brewed coffee
> 1 teaspoon unsweetened cocoa powder
> 1 teaspoon vanilla
> 1 packet sugar substitute *or* equivalent of 2 teaspoons sugar

1. Place all ingredients in food processor or blender; process until smooth. Place container in freezer; freeze 1½ to 2 hours or until top and sides of mixture are partially frozen.

2. Scrape sides of container; process until smooth and frothy. Garnish as desired. Serve immediately.

Iced Mocha Cappuccino: Increase amount of unsweetened cocoa powder to 1 tablespoon. Proceed as above.

Tip: To add an extra flavor boost, add orange peel, lemon peel or a dash of ground cinnamon to your coffee grounds before brewing.

Nutrients per serving:
Calories: 105, **Calories from Fat:** 0%, **Total Fat:** <1g,
Saturated Fat: <1g, **Cholesterol:** <1mg, **Sodium:** 72mg,
Carbohydrate: 21g, **Fiber:** 0g, **Protein:** 5g

Dietary Exchange: 1½ Starch

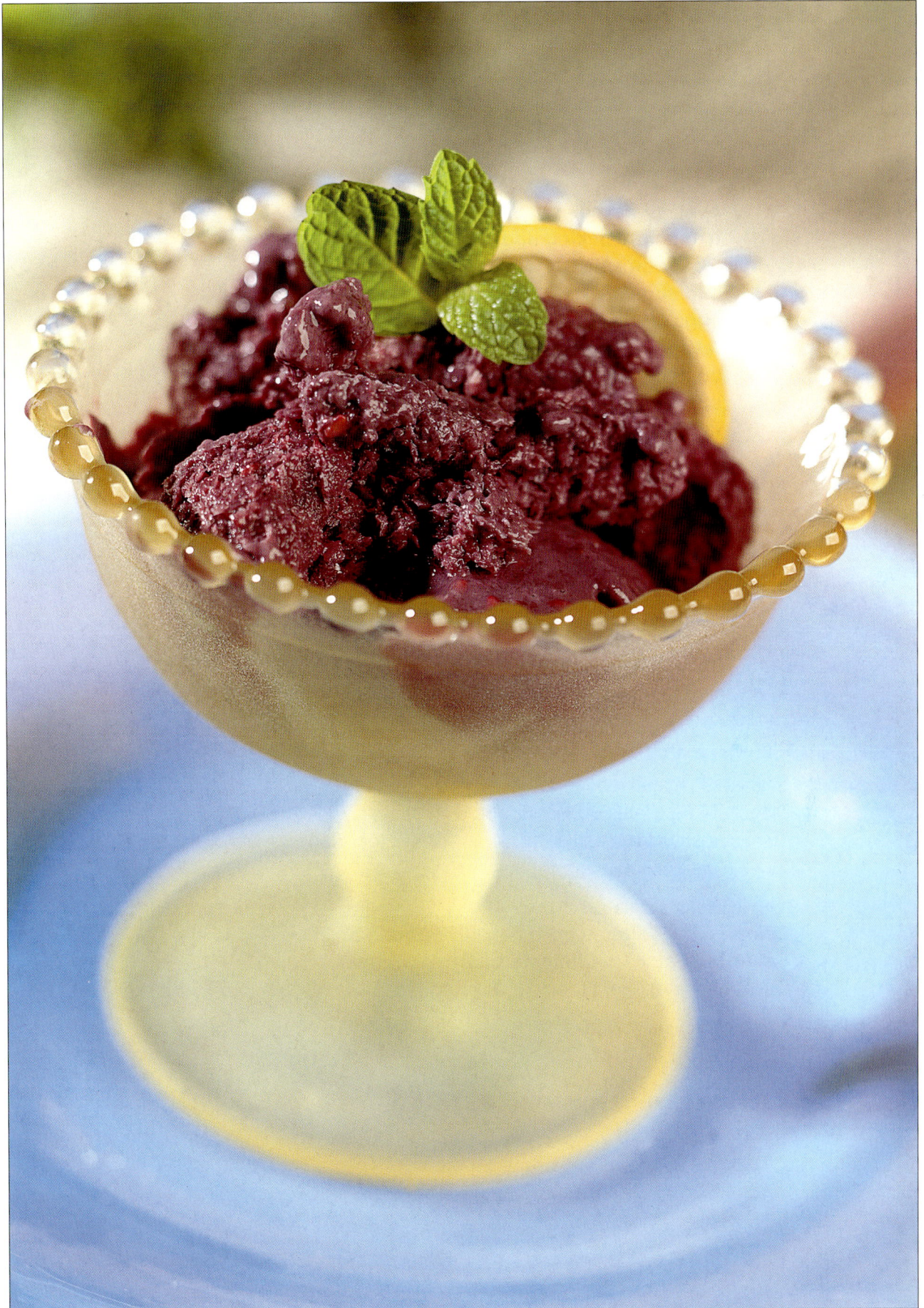

Blackberry Sorbet

Apricot Biscotti

Makes 2½ dozen biscotti

  3 **cups all-purpose flour**
1½ **teaspoons baking soda**
  ½ **teaspoon salt**
  ⅔ **cup sugar**
  3 **eggs**
  1 **teaspoon vanilla**
  ½ **cup chopped dried apricots***
  ⅓ **cup sliced almonds, chopped**
  1 **tablespoon reduced-fat (2%) milk**

*Other chopped dried fruits, such as dried cherries, cranberries or blueberries, can be substituted.

1. Preheat oven to 350°F. Lightly coat cookie sheet with nonstick cooking spray; set aside.

2. Combine flour, baking soda and salt in medium bowl; set aside.

3. Beat sugar, eggs and vanilla in large bowl with electric mixer at medium speed until blended. Add flour mixture; beat until well blended.

4. Stir in apricots and almonds. Turn dough out onto lightly floured work surface. Knead 4 to 6 times. Shape dough into 20-inch log; place on prepared cookie sheet. Brush dough with milk.

5. Bake 30 minutes or until firm. Remove from oven; cool 10 minutes. Diagonally slice into 30 biscotti. Place slices on cookie sheet. Bake 10 minutes; turn and bake additional 10 minutes. Cool on wire racks. Store in airtight container.

Nutrients per serving: 1 cookie
Calories: 86, **Calories from Fat:** 10%, **Total Fat:** 1g,
Saturated Fat: <1g, **Cholesterol:** 21mg, **Sodium:** 108mg,
Carbohydrate: 16g, **Fiber:** 1g, **Protein:** 2g

Dietary Exchange: 1 Starch

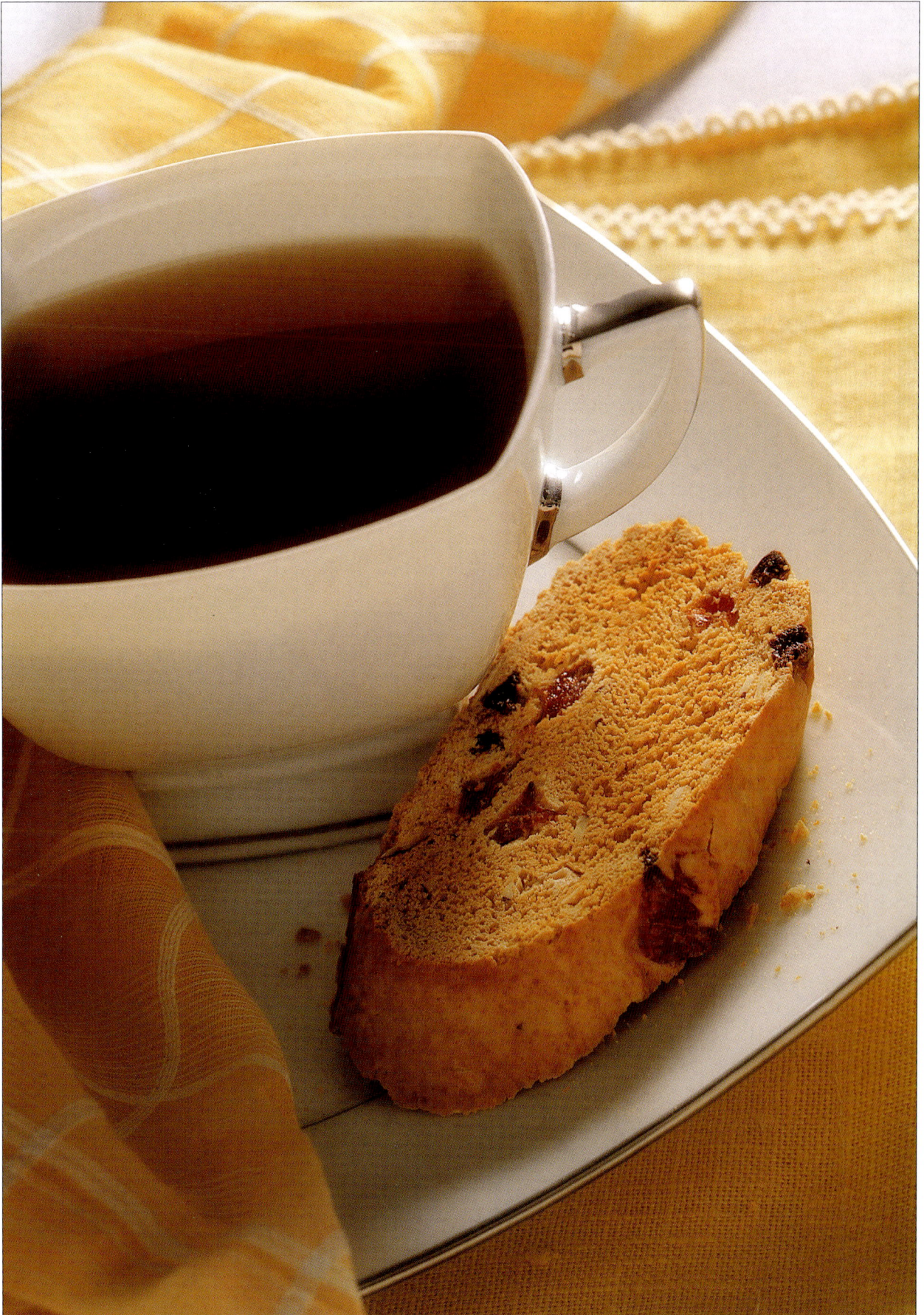

Apricot Biscotti

Mixed Berry Cheesecake

Makes 16 servings

CRUST

- 1½ cups fruit-juice-sweetened breakfast cereal flakes*
- 15 sugar-free low-fat butter-flavored cookies*
- 1 tablespoon vegetable oil

CHEESECAKE

- 2 packages (8 ounces each) fat-free cream cheese, softened
- 2 cartons (8 ounces each) raspberry nonfat yogurt
- 1 package (8 ounces) Neufchâtel cream cheese, softened
- ½ cup no-sugar-added seedless blackberry preserves
- ½ cup no-sugar-added blueberry preserves
- 6 packets sugar substitute *or* equivalent of ¼ cup sugar
- 1 tablespoon vanilla
- ¼ cup water
- 1 package (4-serving size) sugar-free strawberry-flavored gelatin

TOPPING

- 3 cups fresh or frozen unsweetened mixed berries, thawed

Available in the health food section of supermarkets.

1. Preheat oven to 400°F. Spray 10-inch springform pan with nonstick cooking spray.

2. To prepare crust, combine cereal, cookies and oil in food processor; process with on/off pulses until finely crushed. Press firmly onto bottom and ½ inch up side of pan. Bake 5 to 8 minutes or until crust is golden.

3. To prepare cheesecake, combine cream cheese, yogurt, Neufchâtel cheese, preserves, sugar substitute and vanilla in large bowl. Beat with electric mixer at high speed until smooth.

4. Combine water and gelatin in small microwavable bowl; microwave at HIGH 30 seconds to 1 minute or until water is boiling and gelatin is dissolved. Cool slightly. Add to cheese mixture; beat an additional 2 to 3 minutes or until well blended. Pour into prepared pan; cover and refrigerate at least 24 hours. Top cheesecake with berries before serving.

Nutrients per serving: 1 Cheesecake slice (¹⁄₁₆ of total recipe) with 3 tablespoons berries for topping
Calories: 186, **Calories from Fat:** 24%, **Total Fat:** 5g,
Saturated Fat: 2g, **Cholesterol:** 11mg, **Sodium:** 290mg,
Carbohydrate: 26g, **Fiber:** 2g, **Protein:** 8g

Dietary Exchange: ½ Starch, 1½ Fruit, 1 Meat, ½ Fat

Apple-Cranberry Crescent Cookies

Makes 2 dozen cookies

- 1¼ **cups chopped apples**
- ½ **cup dried cranberries**
- ½ **cup reduced-fat sour cream**
- ¼ **cup cholesterol-free egg substitute**
- ¼ **cup (½ stick) margarine or butter, melted**
- 3 **tablespoons sugar, divided**
- 1 **package quick-rise active dry yeast**
- 1 **teaspoon vanilla**
- 2 **cups all-purpose flour**
- 1 **teaspoon ground cinnamon**
- 1 **tablespoon reduced-fat (2%) milk**

1. Preheat oven to 350°F. Lightly coat cookie sheet with nonstick cooking spray.

2. Place apples and cranberries in food processor or blender; process with on/off pulses until finely chopped. Set aside.

3. Combine sour cream, egg substitute, margarine and 2 tablespoons sugar in medium bowl. Add yeast and vanilla. Add flour; stir to form ball. Turn dough out onto lightly floured work surface. Knead 1 minute. Cover with plastic wrap; let stand 10 minutes.

4. Divide dough into thirds. Roll one portion into 12-inch circle. Spread with ⅓ apple mixture (about ¼ cup). Cut dough to make 8 wedges. Roll up each wedge, beginning at outside edge. Place on prepared cookie sheet; turn ends of cookies to form crescents. Repeat with remaining dough and apple mixture.

5. Combine remaining 1 tablespoon sugar and cinnamon in small bowl. Lightly brush cookies with milk; sprinkle with sugar-cinnamon mixture. Bake 18 to 20 minutes or until lightly browned.

Nutrients per serving: 1 Cookie
Calories: 82, **Calories from Fat:** 22%, **Total Fat:** 2g,
Saturated Fat: 1g, **Cholesterol:** 2mg, **Sodium:** 31mg,
Carbohydrate: 13g, **Fiber:** 1g, **Protein:** 2g

Dietary Exchange: 1 Starch

acknowledgments

The publisher would like to thank the companies and organizations listed below for the use of their recipes and photographs in this publication.

Egg Beaters®

Equal® sweetener

Glucerna® is a registered trademark of Abbott Laboratories

Mushroom Information Center

NatraTaste® is a registered trademark of Stadt Corporation

StarKist® Seafood Company

index

METRIC CONVERSION CHART

VOLUME MEASUREMENTS (dry)

⅛ teaspoon = 0.5 mL
¼ teaspoon = 1 mL
½ teaspoon = 2 mL
¾ teaspoon = 4 mL
1 teaspoon = 5 mL
1 tablespoon = 15 mL
2 tablespoons = 30 mL
¼ cup = 60 mL
⅓ cup = 75 mL
½ cup = 125 mL
⅔ cup = 150 mL
¾ cup = 175 mL
1 cup = 250 mL
2 cups = 1 pint = 500 mL
3 cups = 750 mL
4 cups = 1 quart = 1 L

VOLUME MEASUREMENTS (fluid)

1 fluid ounce (2 tablespoons) = 30 mL
4 fluid ounces (½ cup) = 125 mL
8 fluid ounces (1 cup) = 250 mL
12 fluid ounces (1½ cups) = 375 mL
16 fluid ounces (2 cups) = 500 mL

WEIGHTS (mass)

½ ounce = 15 g
1 ounce = 30 g
3 ounces = 90 g
4 ounces = 120 g
8 ounces = 225 g
10 ounces = 285 g
12 ounces = 360 g
16 ounces = 1 pound = 450 g

DIMENSIONS

1/16 inch = 2 mm
⅛ inch = 3 mm
¼ inch = 6 mm
½ inch = 1.5 cm
¾ inch = 2 cm
1 inch = 2.5 cm

OVEN TEMPERATURES

250°F = 120°C
275°F = 140°C
300°F = 150°C
325°F = 160°C
350°F = 180°C
375°F = 190°C
400°F = 200°C
425°F = 220°C
450°F = 230°C

BAKING PAN SIZES

Utensil	Size in Inches/Quarts	Metric Volume	Size in Centimeters
Baking or Cake Pan (square or rectangular)	8×8×2	2 L	20×20×5
	9×9×2	2.5 L	23×23×5
	12×8×2	3 L	30×20×5
	13×9×2	3.5 L	33×23×5
Loaf Pan	8×4×3	1.5 L	20×10×7
	9×5×3	2 L	23×13×7
Round Layer Cake Pan	8×1½	1.2 L	20×4
	9×1½	1.5 L	23×4
Pie Plate	8×1¼	750 mL	20×3
	9×1¼	1 L	23×3
Baking Dish or Casserole	1 quart	1 L	—
	1½ quart	1.5 L	—
	2 quart	2 L	—